FASTING TO FIT

Your Beginner's Guide on Intermittent Fasting for Optimal Health, Weight Loss, and Aging Slowly with a 4-Week Meal Plan

ALEXIS   JOHNSON

DEDICATION

This book is dedicated to all those who dare to embark on the journey to transform their health and well-being. May your determination, perseverance, and commitment lead you to a life filled with vitality, joy, and fulfillment. Remember, every step you take towards better health is a step towards a brighter future. This book is for

CONTENT

ABOUT THIS BOOK

Unlock the secrets to optimal health, efficient weight loss, and slow aging with "FASTING TO FIT." This comprehensive guide is the ultimate resource for anyone looking to harness the power of intermittent fasting to transform their lives. Here are 10 reasons why this book stands out as the best in its class:

Comprehensive Guide: "FASTING TO FIT" provides a complete overview of intermittent fasting, covering everything from the science behind it to practical tips for implementation.

Expert Guidance: Written by experts in the field of nutrition and wellness, this book offers trusted advice backed by scientific research and real-world experience.

Clear and Concise: Say goodbye to confusing jargon and complicated terminology. "FASTING TO FIT" is written in simple language that anyone can understand, making it accessible to beginners and experts alike.

Proven Strategies: Discover proven strategies for maximizing the benefits of intermittent fasting, including tips for weight loss, improved metabolic health, and enhanced brain function.

Customizable Plans: Whether you're a busy professional or a stay-at-home parent, "FASTING TO FIT" offers customizable fasting plans to fit your lifestyle and goals.

Practical Tips: From meal planning to navigating social situations, this book is packed with practical tips and advice to help you succeed on your fasting journey.

Fasting Journal: Keep track of your progress with the included fasting journal, complete with daily prompts and reflections to help you stay motivated and accountable.

Inspiring Success Stories: Learn from real-life success stories of individuals who have transformed their health and lives through intermittent fasting. Their stories will inspire and motivate you to achieve your own goals.

Holistic Approach: "FASTING TO FIT" takes a holistic approach to health and wellness, addressing not only physical health but also mental and emotional well-being.

Life-Changing Results: Whether you're looking to lose weight, boost energy levels, or slow down the aging process, "FASTING TO FIT" has the tools and strategies you need to achieve life-changing results.

Don't settle for mediocrity when it comes to your health. With "FASTING TO FIT," you have the ultimate guide to unlocking your full potential and living your best life. Are you ready to transform your health and embrace a new way of living? Start your journey today.

INTRODUCTION

Welcome to "Fasting to Fit," where we're about to embark on a journey toward a healthier lifestyle through the power of intermittent fasting. If you've ever felt frustrated with traditional diets or overwhelmed by complicated fitness plans, you're in the right place.

Let me introduce myself: I'm Alexis Johnson, and I used to struggle with my weight and overall health. Like many of you, I tried every diet under the sun, from low carb to juice cleanses, with little success. It wasn't until I discovered intermittent fasting that everything changed for me.

Picture this: I was tired of feeling sluggish and uncomfortable in my own skin. I wanted to be active and energetic, but my unhealthy habits were holding me back. That's when a friend introduced me to intermittent fasting. At first, I was skeptical. Skipping meals? How could that possibly lead to weight loss and better health?

But I decided to give it a try, and I'm so glad I did. Not only did I shed those stubborn pounds, but I also experienced a whole range of unexpected benefits. My energy levels skyrocketed, my cravings became more manageable, and I even noticed improvements in my mood and mental clarity.

Through my own journey, I've learned that intermittent fasting is more than just a fad diet—it's a sustainable lifestyle approach that can truly transform your health from the inside out. And now, I'm excited to share everything I've learned with you.

In this book, we'll dive deep into the science behind intermittent fasting, explore different fasting methods, and uncover the incredible benefits it can offer. But more importantly, we'll discuss practical strategies for getting started, staying motivated, and overcoming common challenges along the way.

Whether you're looking to lose weight, boost your energy, or simply improve your overall well-being, intermittent fasting can be the tool you need to achieve your goals. So, are you ready to join me on this journey to a healthier, happier you? Let's dive in and discover the transformative power of fasting together.

In the pages that follow, we'll break down the sometimes-complex world of intermittent fasting into easy-to-understand concepts and practical tips. But before we dive into the nitty-gritty details, let's take a moment to understand what intermittent fasting is all about.

To put it simply, intermittent fasting is a pattern of eating those alternates between eating and fasting intervals. It's not about depriving yourself of food or counting every calorie. Instead, it's about changing when you eat to optimize your body's natural rhythms and improve your health.

Now, you might be wondering: How does intermittent fasting work? Well, that's what we'll explore in the coming chapters. We'll delve into the science behind fasting and uncover how it affects your metabolism, hormones, and overall well-being.

But perhaps the most exciting part of intermittent fasting is its potential to transform your life in ways you never imagined. From weight loss and improved metabolic health to enhanced brain function and longevity, the benefits of fasting are truly remarkable.

And the best part? Intermittent fasting is not a one-size-fits-all approach. There are various fasting methods to choose from, allowing you to find the one that fits your lifestyle and preferences. Whether you prefer the simplicity of the 16/8 method or the flexibility of the 5:2 diet, there's a fasting protocol that's right for you.

But intermittent fasting is more than just a diet—it's a lifestyle. It's about embracing a new way of eating that nourishes your body and nourishes your soul. It's about listening to your body's cues, honoring its needs, and finding balance in all aspects of your life.

As we embark on this journey together, it's important to remember that change doesn't happen overnight. It takes time, patience, and commitment. But trust me when I say that the rewards are well worth the effort.

Throughout the pages of "Fasting to Fit," you'll find everything you need to know to make intermittent fasting a sustainable and rewarding part of your life. From practical tips on meal planning and managing cravings to strategies for overcoming common challenges and staying motivated, I've got you covered.

But remember, the journey doesn't end when you close this book. It's just the beginning. The real magic happens when you take what you've learned and put it into practice in your everyday life. So, don't be afraid to experiment, to make mistakes, and to learn from them.

And whenever you need a little extra support or guidance, know that I'm here for you. Whether it's through the pages of this book, our online community, or a simple email, I'm committed to helping you achieve your health and wellness goals.

let's make a pact right now: no matter where you are on your journey, no matter how many obstacles you face, we'll tackle them together. We'll celebrate your successes, learn from your setbacks, and grow stronger with each passing day.

So, are you ready to work the work with me? Are you ready to take control of your health, transform your body, and unleash your full potential? If so, then let's dive in and make "Fasting to Fit" the start of something truly amazing.

Here is to a healthier and happier you!

PART ONE

The Basics of Intermittent Fasting

What is Intermittent Fasting

Intermittent fasting is like a special way of eating where you don't eat for a certain time and then eat during another time. It's not about what you eat, but when you eat.

What is Intermittent Fasting?

A method of eating called intermittent fasting involves alternating between eating and fasting intervals. It's not about counting calories or following complicated meal plans. Instead, it's all about when you eat.

When you're fasting, you're not eating any food. You might think that sounds hard, but it's not as tough as it sounds. There are different ways to do intermittent fasting, and you can choose the one that works best for you.

One popular method is the 16/8 method. This implies you have an 8-hour window for eating and a 16-hour fast. For example, you might stop eating at 8 p.m. and wait till noon the following day to eat again. Another method is the 5:2 diet, where you eat normally for five days of the week and then eat very few calories (about 500-600) on the other two days.

So why would anyone want to fast? Well, there are a bunch of benefits that come with intermittent fasting. It can help you lose weight, improve your metabolic health, and even boost your brain function.

History and Evolution of Fasting

Fasting isn't a new idea. In fact, people have been fasting for thousands of years for all sorts of reasons. In ancient times, fasting was often used for religious or spiritual purposes. People believed that fasting could cleanse the body and purify the soul.

But fasting wasn't just about religion. The body was also healed with it. Ancient healers believed that fasting could help cure all sorts of ailments, from fevers to digestive issues.

Today, fasting is more popular than ever. People all over the world are turning to intermittent fasting to improve their health and lose weight. And with all the scientific research backing up its benefits, it's no wonder why.

The Science Behind Intermittent Fasting

So why does intermittent fasting work? It all comes down to how our bodies are designed to function.

When you eat food, your body breaks it down into glucose, which is a type of sugar that your cells use for energy. Any extra glucose that your body doesn't need right away gets stored in your liver and muscles for later.

But what happens when you're not eating? Your body still needs energy to function, so it starts burning fat instead. This is what makes intermittent fasting such an effective way to lose weight. By giving your body a break from eating, you force it to burn fat for fuel instead of relying on the food you eat all the time.

But weight loss is just the beginning. Intermittent fasting has a whole bunch of other benefits too. It can improve your metabolic health by reducing insulin resistance and lowering blood sugar levels. It can also help protect against diseases like heart disease, cancer, and Alzheimer's.

So, there you have it. Intermittent fasting might sound like a fancy new trend, but it's just a simple way to give your body a break from eating. And with all the benefits it offers, it's worth giving it a try.

Different Methods of Intermittent Fasting

Intermittent fasting, or IF for short, is all about giving your body a break from eating for a certain period. However, did you realize that there are other approaches? That's right! Whether you're new to fasting or looking to switch things up, there's a method that's right for you. Let's take a closer look at some simple intermittent fasting methods:

1. 16/8 Method:
The 16/8 method is one of the most popular and straightforward ways to do intermittent fasting. Here's how it works: you fast for 16 hours each day and eat during an 8-hour window. For instance, you may decide to eat between 12 p.m. and 8 p.m. and fast from 8 p.m. until 12 p.m. the next day.

This method is great for beginners because it's easy to follow and doesn't require any special equipment or expensive ingredients. Plus, you still get to enjoy all your favorite foods during your eating window!

During the fasting period, your body starts burning fat for energy instead of relying on food you eat all the time. This can help you lose weight without feeling hungry all the time. Plus, fasting has been shown to have other health benefits, like improving your metabolism, regulating your blood sugar levels, and even enhancing brain function.

2. 5:2 Diet:
The 5:2 diet is another popular intermittent fasting method that's super simple to follow. With this method, you eat normally for five days of the week and then restrict your calories to about 500-600 calories per day for the remaining two days.

On your fasting days, you might choose to eat smaller meals throughout the day or have one larger meal. It's up to you! The key is to stick to your calorie limit and avoid overeating.

This method is great for people who don't want to completely give up their favorite foods but still want to see results. Plus, it's flexible enough to fit into any schedule.

Fasting for two days a week might sound challenging, but many people find that it gets easier over time. And the best part? You still get to enjoy all your favorite foods on your non-fasting days!

3. Eat-Stop-Eat:
Eat-stop-eat is a slightly more advanced intermittent fasting method that involves fasting for 24 hours once or twice a week.

You may decide, for instance, to fast from supper on one day until dinner on the next day.

During the fasting period, you can drink water, tea, or coffee to help curb hunger. Some people also find it helpful to keep busy and distracted during this time to take their minds off food.

This method is great for people who want to see fast results and are willing to put in a little extra effort. Fasting for 24 hours might sound daunting, but many people find that it gets easier with practice.

Plus, the longer fasting period allows your body to enter a state called ketosis, where it starts burning fat for energy instead of glucose. This can lead to faster weight loss and other health benefits, like improved insulin sensitivity and reduced inflammation.

4. Alternate-Day Fasting:
Alternate-day fasting is exactly what it sounds like: you alternate between fasting days and non-fasting days. On fasting days, you restrict your calorie intake to about 500-600 calories, while on non-fasting days, you eat normally.

This method is great for people who like structure and routine. Plus, it's flexible enough to fit into any lifestyle.

Some people find it helpful to plan their fasting days around their schedule, like fasting on weekdays and eating normally on weekends. Others prefer to alternate fasting days throughout the week. It's up to you!

Alternate-day fasting has been shown to be just as effective as daily calorie restriction for weight loss and other health benefits. Plus, it can be easier to stick to long-term because you don't have to completely give up your favorite foods.

5. OMAD (One Meal a Day):
OMAD, or one meal a day, is one of the simplest intermittent fasting methods out there. As the name suggests, you eat just one meal a day and fast for the remaining 23 hours.

This method is great for people who want to simplify their eating habits and don't mind eating large meals. Plus, it can be a time-saver because you don't have to worry about planning or preparing multiple meals throughout the day.

Some people find it helpful to eat their one meal at the same time every day to create a routine. Others prefer to be more flexible and eat whenever they feel hungry. It's up to you!

OMAD has been shown to be just as effective as other intermittent fasting methods for weight loss and other health benefits. Plus, it can help improve your relationship with food and break the cycle of constant snacking.

intermittent fasting doesn't have to be complicated. With simple methods like the 16/8 method, 5:2 diet, eat-stop-eat, alternate-day fasting, and OMAD, you can reap the benefits of fasting without all the hassle. So why not give it a try? Your body will thank you for it!

Benefits of Intermittent Fasting

In a world filled with endless dieting trends and health fads, one approach stands out for its simplicity and effectiveness: intermittent fasting. This straightforward eating pattern involves cycling between periods of eating and fasting, with no need for complex meal plans or calorie counting. Instead, it's about giving your body a break from eating for a certain period of time. What makes intermittent fasting truly remarkable are the incredible benefits it offers, touching every aspect of our health and well-being. And guess what? This simple change can bring a whole bunch of benefits that can make a big difference in your life.

Let's break it down and make it super simple:

1. Weight Loss:

Have you ever wanted to lose weight without feeling hungry all the time? Intermittent fasting might be just what you need. When you fast, your body starts burning fat for energy instead of relying on food you eat all the time. This can help you shed those extra pounds without feeling like you're starving yourself. Let me share my own experience with you. Like many others, I struggled with my weight for years, trying every diet under the sun with little success. Then I discovered intermittent fasting. By simply restricting my eating to a specific window of time each day, I started shedding pounds effortlessly. No more constantly worrying about what I was eating or feeling guilty about indulging in my favorite foods. Intermittent fasting made weight loss feel like a natural part of my daily routine.

2. Improved Metabolic Health:

Your metabolism is like the engine that keeps your body running smoothly. Intermittent fasting can help improve your metabolism by giving it a little tune-up. It can help regulate your blood sugar levels, lower your cholesterol, and even reduce inflammation in your body. All of these things can add up to better overall health. Before, I struggled with high cholesterol and unstable blood sugar levels. But with intermittent fasting, my body became more efficient at processing nutrients and regulating my metabolism. My cholesterol levels improved, my blood sugar stabilized, and I felt more energized throughout the day. It was like giving my body a much-needed tune-up.

3. Enhanced Brain Function:

One of the most surprising benefits of intermittent fasting was its impact on my brain function. I used to struggle with brain fog and difficulty concentrating, especially in the afternoons. But after incorporating intermittent fasting into my routine, I noticed a remarkable improvement in my mental clarity and focus. I felt sharper and more alert throughout the day, making it easier to tackle tasks and stay productive. It was like giving my brain a boost of energy whenever I needed it most. Ever feel like your brain is a little foggy? Intermittent fasting might be able to help clear that fog away. When you fast, your brain produces more of a protein called brain-derived neurotrophic factor (BDNF). This protein helps your brain grow new neurons and strengthens the connections between them. The result? Better memory, sharper focus, and improved cognitive function.

4. Longevity and Aging:

Who doesn't want to live a long and healthy life? Intermittent fasting might hold the key to unlocking the fountain of youth. Studies have shown that fasting can help extend your lifespan by protecting your cells from damage and reducing the risk of age-related diseases like heart disease, cancer, and Alzheimer's. As I continued my intermittent fasting journey, I started to notice another unexpected benefit: a slower aging process. Studies have shown that intermittent fasting can help protect against age-related diseases and extend lifespan. By promoting cellular repair and reducing inflammation, intermittent fasting has the potential to keep us looking and feeling younger for longer. It's like hitting the pause button on the aging process and giving our bodies a chance to rejuvenate from the inside out.

5. Hormonal Balance:

Hormones are like little messengers that tell your body what to do. When your hormones are out of whack, it can throw everything off balance. Maintaining hormonal balance is crucial for overall health and well-being, and intermittent fasting can help with that too. I used to struggle with hormonal imbalances that left me feeling moody and fatigued. But with intermittent fasting, my hormones became more balanced, leading to improved mood, better sleep, and increased energy levels. It was like finding the missing piece of the puzzle that finally brought everything into harmony. Intermittent fasting can help regulate your hormones, including insulin, cortisol, and growth hormone. This can lead to better energy levels, improved mood, and even better sleep.

6. Disease Prevention:
Nobody wants to get sick, right? Perhaps the most compelling benefit of intermittent fasting is its potential to prevent chronic diseases. Heart disease, diabetes, cancer – these are all too common in today's society, but they don't have to be our destiny. By reducing inflammation, improving insulin sensitivity, and promoting cellular repair, intermittent fasting can help lower our risk of developing these serious health conditions. It's like giving our bodies the ultimate form of protection from the inside out.

So, there you have it, folk. Intermittent fasting might sound fancy, but it's just a simple way to give your body a little break from eating. And the best part? It comes with lots of amazing benefits. In conclusion, intermittent fasting is not just a diet; it's a lifestyle change that can revolutionize your health and well-being. From weight loss to improved metabolic health, enhanced brain function, longevity, hormonal balance, and disease prevention, the benefits are undeniable. So why not give it a try? Start small, experiment with different fasting protocols, and see how your body responds. You might just be amazed at the transformation that awaits you that can help you look and feel your best. Your body will thank you for it!

PART TWO

Getting Started with Intermittent Fasting

Getting ready to start something new can be both exciting and a little scary. Whether it's taking up a new hobby, starting a new job, or embarking on a journey like intermittent fasting, preparation is key. we'll explore the importance of preparing yourself mentally and physically for the journey ahead, sharing personal stories along the way.

Mental Preparation:

Understanding Your Why:

Before diving into any new endeavor, it's crucial to understand why you're doing it. What motivates you to start intermittent fasting? Is it to lose weight, improve your health, or boost your energy levels? Understanding your "why" can give you the mental clarity and determination needed to stay committed when challenges arise.

When I decided to try intermittent fasting, my main motivation was to regain control of my health. After struggling with weight gain and low energy for years, I knew I needed to make a change. Understanding my why gave me the strength to push through the initial discomfort of fasting and stay focused on my goals.

Setting Realistic Expectations:

It's easy to get caught up in the hype surrounding intermittent fasting and expect instant results. However, it's essential to set realistic expectations and understand that progress takes time. Rome wasn't built in a day, and neither will your health transformation.

When I first started intermittent fasting, I expected to see dramatic changes in my weight and energy levels within a week. However, as I soon realized, progress was gradual. By setting realistic expectations and focusing on small victories along the way, I was able to stay motivated and committed to my fasting routine.

Building a Support System:

Starting any new journey is easier when you have a support system cheering you on. Surround yourself with friends, family, or online communities who understand your goals and can offer encouragement when you need it most.

I'll never forget the first time I shared my intermittent fasting journey with a close friend. Instead of skepticism or criticism, they offered unwavering support and even decided to join me on the journey. Having someone to share my successes and struggles with made the experience feel less daunting and more enjoyable.

Physical Preparation:

Consulting with a Healthcare Professional:

Before making any significant changes to your diet or lifestyle, it's essential to consult with a healthcare professional. They can assess your current health status, provide personalized recommendations, and ensure that intermittent fasting is safe for you.

Prior to starting intermittent fasting, I scheduled a visit with my doctor to discuss my plans. They conducted a thorough health assessment, including blood tests and a physical examination, to ensure that I was healthy enough to fast safely. Their approval gave me the confidence to proceed with my fasting journey.

Gradually Adjusting Your Eating Patterns:

Intermittent fasting involves shifting from regular meal patterns to periods of fasting and eating. Instead of diving headfirst into a strict fasting schedule, it's helpful to gradually adjust your eating patterns to allow your body to adapt.

To ease into intermittent fasting, I started by delaying my breakfast by an hour each day until I reached my desired fasting window. This gradual approach allowed my body to adjust to the new eating schedule without feeling overwhelmed or deprived.

Stocking Up on Nutrient-Dense Foods:
During your eating windows, it's essential to nourish your body with nutrient-dense foods that provide the energy and nutrients it needs to thrive. Stock your kitchen with plenty of fruits, vegetables, lean proteins, and whole grains to support your fasting journey.

When I first started intermittent fasting, I made a conscious effort to revamp my pantry and fridge with nutritious foods. Instead of reaching for processed snacks or sugary treats during my eating windows, I stocked up on fresh produce, lean meats, and whole grains. Not only did this improve my overall health, but it also made sticking to my fasting routine easier.

preparing yourself mentally and physically is essential for success on your intermittent fasting journey. By understanding your motivations, setting realistic expectations, building a support system, consulting with healthcare professionals, gradually adjusting your eating patterns, and stocking up on nutrient-dense foods, you'll be well-equipped to embark on this transformative experience. Remember, Rome wasn't built in a day, but with patience, persistence, and preparation, you can achieve your health and wellness goals with intermittent fasting.

Setting Realistic Goals

Setting realistic goals is like drawing a map for your journey. You need to know where you're going and how you're going to get there. When it comes to intermittent fasting, it's important to set goals that are achievable and sustainable. Here's how you can do it:

First, think about what you want to achieve with intermittent fasting. Is it weight loss, better health, or more energy? Once you've figured that out, break your goal down into smaller, manageable steps. For example, if your goal is to lose 20 pounds, aim to lose 1-2 pounds per week.

Make sure your objectives are quantifiable and defined after that. Instead of saying "I want to lose weight," say "I want to lose 10 pounds in the next two months." This way, you'll know exactly what you're working towards and how you'll track your progress.

It's also important to be realistic about your goals. Don't expect to lose 10 pounds in a week or completely overhaul your diet overnight. Rome wasn't built in a day, and neither is a healthy lifestyle. Start small and build from there.

Finally, be flexible with your goals. Life happens, and sometimes things don't go according to plan. If you have a setback, don't beat yourself up about it. Instead, reassess your goals and adjust your plan as needed.

Practical Questionnaire:

1. What are your main goals with intermittent fasting?
2. Have you broken down your goals into smaller, manageable steps?
3. Are your goals specific and measurable?
4. Are your goals realistic given your current lifestyle and commitments?
5. How will you adjust your goals if you encounter setbacks?

Planning Your Fasting Schedule

Planning your fasting schedule is like creating a roadmap for your day. It helps you stay on track and ensures that you're getting the most out of your fasting experience. Here's how you can do it:

First, decide which fasting method works best for you. There are many different methods to choose from, including the 16/8 method, the 5:2 diet, and alternate day fasting. Experiment with different methods and see which one fits your lifestyle and preferences.

Once you've chosen a fasting method, it's time to plan your fasting schedule. Decide when you'll start and end your fasting period each day and stick to it as much as possible. For intermittent fasting to be effective, consistency is key.

It's also important to listen to your body and adjust your fasting schedule as needed. If you're feeling overly hungry or tired, it's okay to break your fast early or take a day off from fasting altogether. Remember, intermittent fasting is meant to be flexible and sustainable.

Finally, be patient with yourself as you adjust to your new fasting schedule. It may take some time for your body to adapt, so don't be discouraged if you don't see results right away. Keep experimenting and tweaking your schedule until you find what works best for you.

Practical Questionnaire:

1. Which fasting method do you plan to follow?
2. Have you decided on your fasting and eating windows?
3. How will you ensure consistency with your fasting schedule?
4. Are you open to adjusting your fasting schedule based on how you feel?
5. How will you track your progress and make changes to your schedule as needed?

Understanding Hunger and Cravings

Understanding hunger and cravings is like learning to speak your body's language. It can help you make better choices and stick to your fasting goals. Here's what you need to know:

First, it's important to understand the difference between hunger and cravings. Hunger is your body's way of signaling that it needs fuel, while cravings are more psychological and often triggered by emotions or environmental cues. Learning to distinguish between the two can help you make more informed decisions about when to eat and when to fast.

Next, pay attention to your body's hunger cues and learn to trust them. Eat when you're truly hungry and stop when you're satisfied. Avoid eating out of boredom, stress, or habit, as this can lead to overeating and derail your fasting goals.

When cravings strike, try to identify the underlying cause. Are you hungry, or are you just craving a certain food out of habit or emotion? If it's the latter, try to find healthier ways to satisfy your cravings, such as going for a walk, drinking water, or distracting yourself with a hobby.

It's also important to nourish your body with nutritious foods during your eating windows. Focus on whole, nutrient-dense foods like fruits, vegetables, lean proteins, and healthy fats. This will help keep you satisfied and energized throughout the day.

Finally, remember that it's okay to indulge in your favorite foods occasionally. Intermittent fasting is all about balance and moderation, so don't beat yourself up if you slip up from time to time. The key is to get back on track and keep moving forward.

Practical Questionnaire:

1. How would you describe the difference between hunger and cravings?
2. Are you able to recognize your body's hunger cues?
3. How do you plan to address cravings when they arise?
4. What strategies will you use to ensure you're eating nutritious foods during your eating windows?
5. How will you maintain balance and moderation when it comes to indulging in your favorite foods?

Managing Your Diet During Eating Windows

Managing your diet during eating windows is like being the captain of your own ship. It's up to you to steer it in the right direction and make choices that support your health and well-being. Here's how you can do it:

First, focus on nutrient-dense foods that will fuel your body and keep you feeling satisfied. This means choosing foods that are rich in vitamins, minerals, and other essential nutrients, such as fruits, vegetables, whole grains, lean proteins, and healthy fats.

Next, pay attention to portion sizes and practice mindful eating. Take the time to savor your food and pay attention to how it makes you feel. Eat slowly, chew your food thoroughly, and stop when you're satisfied, rather than when you're stuffed.

It's also important to stay hydrated during your eating windows. Drink plenty of water throughout the day to help keep your body hydrated and support your overall health. You can also enjoy other beverages like herbal tea, sparkling water, or black coffee, but be mindful of added sugars and calories.

When it comes to snacks and treats, aim for balance and moderation. It's okay to indulge in your favorite foods occasionally but try to keep them in check and avoid overdoing it. Choose healthier options whenever possible, such as fresh fruit, nuts, or yogurt, and save indulgent treats for special occasions.

Finally, listen to your body and honor its cues. If you're hungry, eat. If you're full, stop. Trust that your body knows what it needs and make choices that support its health and well-being.

Practical Questionnaire:

1. What types of nutrient-dense foods do you plan to include in your eating windows?
2. How will you practice mindful eating and pay attention to portion sizes?
3. What strategies will you use to stay hydrated during your eating windows?
4. How will you approach snacks and treats while intermittent fasting?
5. How do you plan to listen to your body's cues and make choices that support its health and well-being?

Staying Hydrated During Fasting Periods

Staying hydrated during fasting periods is like giving your body a big drink of water when it's thirsty. It helps keep everything running smoothly and ensures that you feel your best throughout the day. Here's how you can do it:

First, make water your best friend. It's calorie-free, sugar-free, and essential for your body's overall health and well-being. Aim to drink at least 8 glasses of water per day, or more if you're active or live in a hot climate.

If you find plain water boring, try adding a squeeze of lemon or lime for flavor, or infuse it with fresh herbs or fruit. You can also enjoy other hydrating beverages like herbal tea, sparkling water, or black coffee, but be mindful of added sugars and calories.

It's also important to pay attention to your body's thirst cues and drink water throughout the day, even when you're not feeling thirsty. Dehydration can lead to headaches, fatigue, and other unpleasant symptoms, so make sure you're staying on top of your fluid intake.

If you're fasting for an extended period, such as during a longer fast or a water fast, it's especially important to stay hydrated. Drink water regularly throughout the day to help keep your body hydrated and support your overall health and well-being.

Finally, listen to your body and adjust your fluid intake as needed. Everyone's hydration needs are different, so pay attention to how you feel and make sure you're getting enough fluids to keep you feeling your best.

Practical Questionnaire:

1. How much water do you plan to drink per day?
2. What strategies will you use to make sure you're drinking enough water throughout the day?
3. Are there any flavored or infused water options you'd like to try?
4. How will you stay hydrated during fasting periods?
5. How do you plan to listen to your body's thirst cues and adjust your fluid intake as needed?

mastering the art of intermittent fasting requires attention to detail and a commitment to your health and well-being. Setting realistic goals, planning your fasting schedule, understanding hunger and cravings, managing your diet during eating windows, and staying hydrated during fasting periods are all key components of a successful fasting journey.

By setting realistic goals, breaking them down into manageable steps, and staying flexible in your approach, you can set yourself up for success and avoid feeling overwhelmed. Planning your fasting schedule and listening to your body's cues will help you stay on track and make the most of your fasting experience.

Understanding hunger and cravings and managing your diet during eating windows are crucial for maintaining balance and moderation. By choosing nutrient-dense foods, practicing mindful eating, and staying hydrated, you can support your body's overall health and well-being while intermittent fasting.

Remember, intermittent fasting is not a one-size-fits-all approach, and what works for one person may not work for another. It's important to experiment, listen to your body, and adjust as needed to find what works best for you.

With patience, perseverance, and a willingness to learn, you can harness the power of intermittent fasting to achieve your health and wellness goals and live your best life.

Keep pushing forward, stay focused on your goals, and never underestimate the power of simplicity when it comes to achieving success with intermittent fasting.

Here's to your health and happiness on your fasting journey!

PART THREE

Maximizing Results with Intermittent Fasting

Combining Intermittent Fasting with Exercise

Are you prepared to reach new heights in terms of fitness and health? Combining intermittent fasting with exercise might just be the secret sauce you've been looking for. It's not about spending hours at the gym or following complicated workout routines. Instead, it's about making simple changes to your daily routine that can have a big impact on your overall health and fitness.

Allow me to dissect and simplify it:

Intermittent fasting is a way of eating that involves cycling between periods of eating and fasting. Instead of eating throughout the day, you restrict you're eating to a specific window of time, usually between 8 to 10 hours. The rest of the time, you fast, which means you don't eat any food.

How Does Exercise Fit In?

Exercise is like the cherry on top of the intermittent fasting cake. When you combine intermittent fasting with exercise, you're giving your body a one-two punch that can supercharge your results. Exercise helps you burn more calories, build muscle, and improve your overall fitness levels.

Advantages of Intermittent Fasting and Exercise Together:

Increased Fat Burning: When you exercise in a fasted state, your body must rely on stored fat for energy since there's no food available. This can help you burn fatter and slimmer down faster.

Improved Muscle Growth: Fasting before a workout can also help boost muscle growth. When you exercise in a fasted state, your body produces more growth hormone, which helps stimulate muscle growth and repair.

Enhanced Endurance: Believe it or not, fasting can improve your endurance during exercise. When you fast, your body becomes more efficient at using fat for fuel, which can help you go longer and harder during your workouts.

Better Recovery: Fasting can also help speed up recovery after exercise. By giving your body a break from food, you allow it to focus on repairing and rebuilding muscle tissue, which can help reduce soreness and improve recovery time.

Tips for Combining Intermittent Fasting with Exercise:

Choose the Right Time to Exercise: Some people find it easier to exercise in the morning before breaking their fast, while others prefer to exercise during their eating window. Try out various times to determine which suits you the best.

Stay Hydrated: It's important to stay hydrated, especially when exercising in a fasted state. Drink plenty of water before, during, and after your workout to stay hydrated and prevent dehydration To stay hydrated and avoid dehydration before and after your workout, drink lots of water.

Pay Attention to Your Body: Observe your feelings both during and after your exercise. If you're feeling lightheaded, dizzy, or weak, it may be a sign that you need to adjust your fasting or exercise routine.

Combining intermittent fasting with exercise can be a powerful way to improve your health and fitness. By making simple changes to your daily routine, you can burn fat, build muscle, and improve your overall fitness levels. So why not give it a try? Your body will thank you for it!

Keep in mind that every person is unique, so what works for one person may not work for another. It's crucial to listen to your body and modify as necessary. Experiment with different fasting and exercise routines to find what works best for you. With consistency and dedication, you can achieve your health and fitness goals with intermittent fasting and exercise.

Intermittent Fasting and Muscle Building

Building muscles is like constructing a house; it requires a strong foundation and the right tools. Intermittent fasting might seem like it's at odds with muscle building, but it can complement your efforts and help you achieve your goals.

When you fast, your body goes into a state called "fasting mode." During this time, it starts breaking down stored fat for energy instead of relying on food you eat. But what about your muscles? Don't worry; your body is smarter than you think. It knows that muscles are important, so it does everything it can to protect them.

Intermittent fasting can help preserve muscle mass while you're burning fat. How? Well, when you fast, your body releases more human growth hormone (HGH), which is like a superhero hormone for muscle growth. HGH helps repair and rebuild muscles, so you can bounce back stronger after a workout.

But wait, there's more! Intermittent fasting can also improve your body's insulin sensitivity, which means your muscles can use glucose more efficiently for fuel. This can lead to better performance during workouts and faster recovery times afterward.

So how can you use intermittent fasting to maximize muscle building? It's simple:

Timing is Everything: Plan your fasting periods around your workouts to take advantage of the muscle-building benefits of fasting mode. Some people find that working out in a fasted state can actually enhance their performance and results.

Eat the Right Foods: When you do eat, make sure you're getting plenty of protein to support muscle growth and repair. Lean meats, fish, eggs, and dairy products are all good sources of protein that can help you reach your muscle-building goals.

Keep Yourself Hydrated: Both general health and muscle building depend on drinking lots of water. Aim to drink at least eight glasses of water a day and consider adding electrolytes to your water if you're fasting for extended periods.

Pay Attention to Your Body: Observe how your body reacts to short bursts of fasting and modify your strategy accordingly. If you're feeling fatigued or run down, it might be a sign that you need to tweak your fasting schedule or eat more during your eating windows.

Be Patient: Building muscles takes time, so don't expect to see results overnight. Stick to your fasting and workout routine consistently, and trust that your efforts will pay off in the long run.

In summary, intermittent fasting can be a powerful tool for muscle building when used correctly. By timing your fasts around your workouts, eating the right foods, staying hydrated, listening to your body, and being patient, you can maximize your muscle-building potential and achieve the strong, lean physique you've always wanted.

Intermittent Fasting for Women

Intermittent fasting isn't just for men; it can be equally beneficial for women. However, women may need to approach intermittent fasting differently than men due to differences in hormones and metabolism.

One of the biggest concerns for women when it comes to intermittent fasting is the potential impact on their menstrual cycle and hormonal balance. Some women worry that fasting might disrupt their hormones or lead to irregular periods. While intermittent fasting can affect hormones, especially in the beginning, it's generally considered safe for most women.

Here are some tips for women who want to try intermittent fasting:

Start Slow: If you're new to intermittent fasting, start with shorter fasting periods and gradually increase the length as your body adjusts. This can help minimize any negative side effects and allow your hormones to adapt gradually.

Pay Attention to Your Body: Observe how your body reacts to short bursts of fasting and modify your strategy accordingly. If you notice any negative symptoms like fatigue, irritability, or changes in your menstrual cycle, consider easing up on your fasting schedule or consulting with a healthcare professional.

Consider Your Goals: The type of intermittent fasting that works best for you may depend on your goals and lifestyle. Some women find that shorter fasting windows, such as the 16/8 method, work better for them, while others prefer longer fasting periods. Try out various strategies to determine which one works best for you.

Nourish Your Body: When you do eat, make sure you're getting plenty of nutrient-dense foods to support your overall health and well-being. Focus on eating a balanced diet rich in fruits, vegetables, lean proteins, and healthy fats to ensure you're getting all the nutrients your body needs.

Stay Hydrated: Drinking plenty of water is essential for everyone, but especially for women who are fasting. Aim to drink at least eight glasses of water a day and consider adding electrolytes to your water if you're fasting for extended periods.

Be Patient: Just like with muscle building, it's important to be patient and give your body time to adapt to intermittent fasting. Don't expect to see results overnight and be prepared to adjust your fasting schedule as needed.

In conclusion, intermittent fasting can be a safe and effective way for women to improve their health, lose weight, and achieve their fitness goals. By starting slow, listening to your body, considering your goals, nourishing your body, staying hydrated, and being patient, you can reap the benefits of intermittent fasting while maintaining your hormonal balance and overall well-being.

Dealing with Plateaus and Challenges

Plateaus and challenges are common experiences when embarking on an intermittent fasting journey. It's essential to understand that encountering obstacles along the way is normal and can be overcome with the right mindset and strategies.

Identifying Plateaus: Plateaus occur when your progress stalls, and you stop seeing the results you desire, whether it's weight loss, improved health markers, or other benefits of intermittent fasting. Recognizing when you've hit a plateau is the first step in overcoming it.

Remain Consistent: When it comes to intermittent fasting, consistency is essential. Even when you're not seeing immediate results, sticking to your fasting schedule and healthy eating habits will eventually pay off. Have faith in the process and proceed accordingly.

Reassess Your Approach: If you've hit a plateau, it may be time to reassess your approach to intermittent fasting. Consider whether you need to adjust your fasting schedule, change up your diet, or incorporate different types of exercises to break through the plateau.

Mix Things Up: Sometimes, your body needs a little shake-up to get things moving again. Try incorporating intermittent fasting variations like alternate-day fasting or OMAD (one meal a day) into your routine to challenge your body in new ways.

Focus on Non-Scale Victories: While the number on the scale is one way to measure progress, it's essential to focus on other indicators of success as well. Pay attention to how you feel, your energy levels, your sleep quality, and any improvements in your overall health and well-being.

Practice Patience: Plateaus are temporary setbacks, not permanent roadblocks. Remember that progress takes time, and it's normal to experience ups and downs along the way. Continue focusing on your goals, exercising patience, and working toward them.

Listening to Your Body: Signs to Watch Out For

It's important to pay attention to your body while you practice intermittent fasting. Your body has a way of communicating with you, and it's essential to pay attention to the signals it sends.

Hunger and Fullness: Pay attention to your hunger and fullness cues. While it's normal to experience some hunger during fasting periods, extreme hunger or feelings of deprivation may indicate that you need to adjust your fasting schedule or eat more during your eating windows.

Energy Levels: Pay attention to the variations in your energy levels during the day. Intermittent fasting should leave you feeling energized and focused, not sluggish or fatigued. If you find that fasting is draining your energy, consider whether you need to modify your fasting schedule or eat more nutrient-dense foods to support your body's needs.

Mood and Mental Health: Intermittent fasting should enhance your mood and mental clarity, not leave you feeling irritable or anxious. Pay attention to how fasting affects your mood and mental health and be proactive about taking care of your emotional well-being.

Physical Symptoms: Be mindful of any physical symptoms you experience while fasting, such as headaches, dizziness, or digestive issues. These symptoms may indicate that your body is struggling to adapt to intermittent fasting, and you may need to make adjustments to your approach.

Overall Well-being: Ultimately, the goal of intermittent fasting is to improve your overall health and well-being. Listen to your body's signals and make choices that support your long-term health and happiness.

Common Myths and Misconceptions About Intermittent Fasting

Intermittent fasting has gained popularity in recent years, but along with its rise in popularity comes a fair share of myths and misconceptions. Let's debunk some of the most common myths surrounding intermittent fasting:

Myth: Intermittent fasting is just another fad diet.
Fact: Intermittent fasting is not a diet; it's a pattern of eating that focuses on when you eat rather than what you eat. Unlike fad diets that often promote restrictive eating habits, intermittent fasting can be sustainable and adaptable to individual preferences and lifestyles.

Myth: Intermittent fasting slows down your metabolism.
Fact: While it's normal to experience a temporary decrease in metabolic rate during fasting periods, intermittent fasting does not permanently slow down your metabolism. In fact, some studies have shown that intermittent fasting can increase metabolic rate and improve metabolic health over time.

Myth: Intermittent fasting is only for weight loss.
Fact: While intermittent fasting can be an effective weight loss tool for many people, its benefits extend far beyond just shedding pounds. Intermittent fasting has been shown to

improve metabolic health, enhance brain function, increase energy levels, and promote longevity.

Myth: Intermittent fasting is not safe for women.
Fact: While women may need to approach intermittent fasting differently than men due to differences in hormones and metabolism, it can be safe and effective for women when done correctly. It's essential for women to listen to their bodies, pay attention to any changes in their menstrual cycle or hormonal balance, and consult with a healthcare professional if they have any concerns.

Myth: Intermittent fasting is only for young, healthy individuals.
Fact: Intermittent fasting can benefit people of all ages and health statuses. While it's essential to consider individual needs and health conditions when practicing intermittent fasting, many people, including older adults and those with chronic health conditions, can safely incorporate intermittent fasting into their lifestyle with guidance from a healthcare professional.

In conclusion, intermittent fasting is a flexible and adaptable approach to eating that can offer a wide range of benefits for both men and women. By understanding how to overcome plateaus and challenges, listening to your body's signals, and debunking common myths and misconceptions, you can make the most of your intermittent fasting journey and achieve your health and wellness goals.

Intermittent fasting is a powerful tool that can help you achieve your health and fitness goals, whether you're looking to lose weight, improve metabolic health, or enhance your overall well-being. By understanding the benefits of intermittent fasting, learning how to navigate challenges and plateaus, and debunking common myths and misconceptions, you can make the most of this simple yet effective approach to eating.

Remember, intermittent fasting is not a one-size-fits-all solution, and what works for one person may not work for another. It's essential to listen to your body, pay attention to how you feel, and adjust your approach as needed. Whether you're new to intermittent fasting or have been practicing it for a while, there's always room for growth and improvement.

As you embark on your intermittent fasting journey, remember to be patient and persistent. Rome wasn't built in a day, and neither is your health and fitness. Have faith in the process, maintain your consistency, and acknowledge your accomplishments as you go.

With the right mindset, strategies, and support, intermittent fasting can be a sustainable and enjoyable way to nourish your body, improve your health, and achieve your wellness goals. So why not give it a try? It's something your body will appreciate.

Here's to your health and happiness!

PART FOUR

Lifestyle and Long-Term Maintenance

Integrating Intermittent Fasting into Your Lifestyle

Intermittent fasting is just a simple way of eating that can bring big benefits to your health. And the best part? It's easy to integrate into your everyday life. Let's break it down and see how you can make intermittent fasting work for you.

How to Make Intermittent Fasting a Part of Your Daily Routine

Start Slow:

If you're new to intermittent fasting, don't jump into it all at once. Start by gradually increasing the amount of time you spend fasting. You can begin with a simple 12-hour fast overnight, then slowly extend it to 14 or 16 hours.

Select a Fasting Schedule That Suits Your Needs:

There's no one-size-fits-all approach to intermittent fasting. You can experiment with different fasting schedules to find what works best for your body and lifestyle. Some popular methods include the 16/8 method, where you fast for 16 hours and eat during an 8-hour window, or the 5:2 method, where you eat normally for five days and limit your calories on two non-consecutive days.

Plan Your Meals Ahead:

Planning can make intermittent fasting much easier. Decide when you'll eat your meals during your eating window and prepare them in advance if possible. This can guarantee that you observe your fasting schedule and help avoid impulsive eating.

Stay Hydrated:
During fasting periods, it's important to stay hydrated. Drink plenty of water throughout the day to keep your body functioning properly. You can also enjoy other non-caloric beverages like herbal tea or black coffee to help curb hunger.

Listen to Your Body:
When you fast, pay attention to how your body feels. If you're feeling excessively hungry or tired, it's okay to adjust your fasting schedule or break your fast early. Remember, intermittent fasting is meant to be flexible and sustainable.

Be Flexible:
Life happens, and it's okay to be flexible with your fasting schedule. If you have a special occasion or social event, you can always modify your fasting routine for that day and resume your regular schedule afterwards. Finding a balance that suits you is crucial.

Focus on Nutrient-Dense Foods:
When it's time to eat, make sure to choose nutrient-dense foods that nourish your body. opt for whole foods like fruits, vegetables, lean proteins, and healthy fats to support your overall health and well-being.

Stay Consistent:
When it comes to intermittent fasting, consistency is essential. Stick to your fasting schedule as much as possible, but don't beat yourself up if you slip up occasionally. Remember, it's about progress, not perfection.

Integrating intermittent fasting into your lifestyle doesn't have to be complicated. With a little planning and flexibility, you can make fasting a seamless part of your daily routine. So why not give it a try? Your body will thank you for it!

Socializing and Dining Out While Fasting

Socializing and dining out can be a bit tricky when you're fasting. But with a little planning and some smart choices, you can still enjoy yourself without breaking your fast. Here are some tips to help you navigate social situations while fasting:

Plan: Before you head out, look at the menu online and choose a restaurant that offers fasting-friendly options. Look for dishes that are high in protein and healthy fats, and low in carbs and sugars. This will help keep you full and satisfied without sabotaging your fast.

Communicate with Friends: Let your friends know that you're fasting and explain why it's important to you. Most people will be understanding and supportive once they understand your goals. Plus, having your friends on board can make it easier to stick to your fasting plan.

Be Mindful of Portions: When dining out, it's easy to overeat, especially when you're hungry. Observe serving sizes and pay attention to your body's signals of hunger. Even if there is food left on your plate, you should stop eating when you are satisfied.

Choose Wisely: opt for simple, whole foods whenever possible. Skip the fried appetizers and sugary drinks, and instead choose grilled meats, salads, and vegetables. And don't be afraid to ask for substitutions or modifications to make a dish more fasting-friendly.

Stay Hydrated: Remember to drink plenty of water throughout the meal to stay hydrated and help curb hunger. You can also try sparkling water or herbal tea if you're craving something more flavorful.

Traveling and Fasting: Tips and Tricks

Traveling can disrupt your fasting routine, but with a little creativity and flexibility, you can still fast while on the go. Here are some tips and tricks to help you stay on track with your fasting goals while traveling:

Pack Snacks: Bring along some fasting-friendly snacks like nuts, seeds, jerky, and protein bars to keep hunger at bay during long flights or road trips. You can avoid impulsive eating and feel full until your next meal by keeping healthy options on hand.

Plan: Research restaurants and grocery stores at your destination that offer fasting-friendly options. Look for places that serve grilled meats, salads, and vegetables, and avoid fast food joints and buffets that tempt you with unhealthy choices.

Intermittent Fasting on the Plane: If you're flying, consider extending your fasting window during the flight to avoid the temptation of airplane food and snacks. Pack some herbal tea or black coffee to sip on during the flight and save your first meal for after you've landed.

Stay Active: Use travel as an opportunity to stay active and explore your surroundings. Go for a walk or hike, rent a bike, or swim in the hotel pool to burn off extra calories and keep your metabolism humming along.

Stay Flexible: Remember that it's okay to be flexible with your fasting schedule while traveling. If you need to adjust your eating window or skip a fast altogether, that's perfectly fine. Making decisions based on your intuition and listening to your body is crucial.

Managing Fasting with Work and Family Life

Balancing fasting with work and family life can be challenging, but with some strategic planning and a little bit of flexibility, you can make it work. Here are some tips to help you manage fasting while juggling your busy schedule:

Set Realistic Expectations: Understand that fasting might require some adjustments to your usual routine, and that's okay. Be realistic about what you can achieve and don't put too much pressure on yourself to be perfect.

Communicate with Your Boss and Co-Workers: If you're fasting during work hours, let your boss and co-workers know about your fasting schedule and any potential changes to your lunch or break times. This can help avoid any misunderstandings and ensure that you have the support you need.

Plan Your Meals and Snacks: Take some time at the beginning of each week to plan out your meals and snacks for the week ahead. This can help prevent impulsive eating and ensure that you have healthy options on hand when hunger strikes.

Get Your Family on Board: If you're fasting while caring for a family, involve them in your fasting journey and explain why it's important to you. Encourage them to support you by offering words of encouragement and avoiding tempting you with unhealthy foods.

Be Flexible: Understand that life is unpredictable, and there may be times when you need to adjust your fasting schedule to accommodate unexpected events or obligations. Be flexible and don't beat yourself up if you need to skip a fast or adjust your eating window occasionally.

Creating a Supportive Environment

Creating a supportive environment is key to sticking to your fasting goals and maintaining your long-term success. Here are some tips to help you create a supportive environment that fosters healthy habits and encourages you to stay on track:

Surround Yourself with Like-Minded People: Surround yourself with friends, family, and co-workers who support your fasting goals and understand why it's important to you. Avoid spending time with people who tempt you with unhealthy foods or try to sabotage your efforts.

Join a Fasting Group or Community: Joining a fasting group or community can provide you with encouragement, accountability, and support on your fasting journey. Look for local meet-up groups, online forums, or social media groups where you can connect with others who share your goals and experiences.

Create a Fasting-Friendly Home Environment: Stock your pantry and fridge with fasting-friendly foods like lean proteins, vegetables, fruits, nuts, and seeds. Remove temptations like sugary snacks, processed foods, and unhealthy beverages that can derail your fasting efforts.

Set Up Your Workspace for Success: If you're fasting during work hours, set up your workspace for success by keeping healthy snacks on hand and avoiding tempting treats that may be lurking in the break room or office kitchen.

Practice Self-Care: Taking care of yourself is essential for maintaining your motivation and resilience on your fasting journey. Practice self-care activities like getting enough sleep, managing stress, staying hydrated, and engaging in activities that bring you joy and fulfillment.

Long-Term Maintenance and Sustainability

Congratulations! You've successfully completed your fasting journey and achieved your health and fitness goals. But now what? How do you maintain your progress and ensure that your results are sustainable in the long term? Here are some tips to help you maintain your fasting routine and make healthy habits a permanent part of your lifestyle:

Set Realistic Maintenance Goals: Now that you've reached your initial goals, it's time to set new goals for long-term maintenance. Be realistic about what you can achieve and focus on maintaining your progress rather than striving for perfection.

Find Your Maintenance Routine: Experiment with different fasting schedules and eating patterns to find a routine that works best for you in the long term. You may need to adjust your fasting window or eating window based on your changing needs and preferences.

Stay Consistent: Consistency is key to maintaining your fasting routine and seeing continued results over time. Stick to your fasting schedule as much as possible, even on weekends and holidays, to keep your metabolism humming along and prevent any backsliding.

Monitor Your Progress: Keep track of your progress by monitoring your weight, measurements, and other key metrics regularly. This can help you stay accountable and catch any potential issues before they become major setbacks.

Practice Mindful Eating: Pay attention to what you eat and how it makes you feel by practicing mindful eating. Listen to your body's hunger and fullness cues, and make conscious choices about when, what, and how much you eat.

PART FIVE:

Keeping Track with Your Fasting Journal

Introduction to Your Fasting Journal

Welcome to your fasting journal! If you're new to the world of intermittent fasting, you might be wondering what a fasting journal is and how it can help you on your journey to better health. Well, wonder no more! In this chapter, we'll introduce you to the basics of your fasting journal and show you how to use it to track your progress, stay motivated, and reach your goals.

What is a Fasting Journal?

First things first, let's talk about what exactly a fasting journal is. Simply put, a fasting journal is a tool that you can use to keep track of your fasting schedule, meals, snacks, and how you're feeling throughout the day. It's like a diary, but specifically focused on your fasting journey.

Why Use a Fasting Journal?

You might be thinking, "Why do I need a journal? Can't I just remember what I eat and when I fast? Yes, you could attempt to keep track of everything in your head, but we assure you that this is far more difficult than it seems. A fasting journal makes it easy to see patterns, identify what's working (and what's not), and stay accountable to yourself.

How to Start Your Fasting Journal

Now that you know what a fasting journal is and why it's useful, let's talk about how to get started with your own journal. Here are a few easy actions to do:

Choose Your Journal: You can use any notebook or journal that you like, but it's a good idea to pick one that's small enough to carry around with you and sturdy enough to withstand daily use.

Set Up Your Journal: Start by creating a title page for your journal and adding some personal touches, like your name or a motivational quote. Then, divide your journal into sections for each day of the week or each fasting period, depending on how you prefer to organize your entries.

Record Your Fasting Schedule: The first thing you'll want to do in your journal is record your fasting schedule. Write down the times when you'll be fasting and the times when you'll be eating. This will help you stay on track and avoid accidentally breaking your fast too early.

Track Your Meals and Snacks: Throughout the day, use your journal to record what you eat and drink during your eating windows. Be sure to include the time, the type of food or drink, and how much you consumed. This will give you a clear picture of your eating habits and help you make healthier choices.

Note How You Feel: In addition to tracking your meals, take some time to jot down how you're feeling throughout the day. Are you feeling hungry, tired, or energized? Are you experiencing any cravings or mood swings? By keeping track of your emotions and physical sensations, you can start to identify patterns and triggers that may be affecting your fasting success.

Reflect and Review: At the end of each day or week, take some time to reflect on your journal entries and review your progress. Celebrate your successes, learn from your challenges, and make any adjustments to your fasting schedule or eating habits as needed.

Setting Up Your Fasting Journal

Setting up your fasting journal is essential for success. By organizing your thoughts and tracking your progress, you'll stay motivated and focused on your goals. Here's a detailed look at how to set up your fasting journal:

Choose Your Journal: The first step is selecting a journal that suits your style and preferences. Whether it's a sleek notebook or a colorful diary, make sure it's something you enjoy using and will want to keep with you daily.

Make Sections: Divide your journal into sections to keep everything organized. Consider creating sections for daily journal prompts, progress tracking, troubleshooting, and reflections. Having designated areas for each aspect of your fasting journey will make it easier to navigate and review your entries.

Gather Supplies: Collect all the supplies you'll need to complete your journal, such as pens, markers, stickers, and sticky notes. Having these items readily available will streamline the journaling process and make it more enjoyable.

With your journal set up, you're ready to embark on your fasting journey with clarity and purpose.

Daily Journal Prompts and Reflections

Daily journal prompts and reflections are invaluable tools for staying engaged with your fasting journey. They provide opportunities for self-reflection, gratitude, and goal setting. Here's how to incorporate them into your journal:

Gratitude: Take a moment each day to list three things for which you are thankful. Practicing gratitude can shift your perspective and enhance your overall well-being.

Intentions: Set intentions for the day ahead by outlining what you hope to accomplish with your fasting journey. Whether it's improving your health, losing weight, or increasing your energy levels, clarifying your intentions can help you stay focused and motivated.

Challenges: Reflect on any challenges you encountered during your fast and how you overcame them. By acknowledging and learning from your challenges, you'll develop resilience and confidence in your ability to navigate obstacles.

Successes: Celebrate your successes, no matter how small. Whether you stuck to your fasting schedule, resisted temptation, or achieved a personal milestone, recognizing your achievements will boost your confidence and motivation.

Reflections: Take time to reflect on your progress and how you're feeling physically, mentally, and emotionally. Consider any changes you've noticed in your body or mindset and document them in your journal.

By incorporating these daily prompts and reflections into your journaling routine, you'll deepen your connection with your fasting journey and cultivate a greater sense of awareness and appreciation.

Tracking Progress and Celebrating Successes

Tracking your progress is very important for staying motivated and accountable. By monitoring key metrics and celebrating your successes, you'll stay engaged and inspired on your fasting journey. Here's how to effectively track your progress and celebrate your achievements:

Measurements: Take baseline measurements of your body, including your weight, waist circumference, and body fat percentage. Update these measurements regularly to track changes over time and celebrate your progress.

Weight: Weigh yourself consistently and record your weight in your journal. Tracking your weight fluctuations can provide valuable insights into your fasting journey's effectiveness and help you identify patterns and trends.

Photos: Capture before and after photos to visually document your progress. Comparing photos side by side can highlight the physical changes you've experienced and serve as a powerful reminder of how far you've come.

Food Diary: Keep a detailed food diary to track your eating habits and behaviors during your eating windows. Recording what you eat and drink can help you identify any patterns or triggers that may be impacting your fasting journey and make informed adjustments as needed.

Mood and Energy: Monitor your mood and energy levels throughout the day and note any changes or fluctuations in your journal. Pay attention to how fasting affects your mental clarity, focus, and overall well-being, and celebrate any improvements you experience.

By diligently tracking your progress and celebrating your successes, you'll stay motivated and inspired to continue making positive changes on your fasting journey.

Troubleshooting and Adjusting Your Approach

Navigating challenges and setbacks is a natural part of any journey, including fasting. By anticipating potential obstacles and proactively adjusting your approach, you'll overcome challenges more effectively and stay on track toward your goals. Here's how to troubleshoot common fasting challenges and adapt your approach as needed:

Plateaus: If you hit a weight loss plateau or notice a stall in your progress, don't panic. Plateaus are common and often temporary. Consider adjusting your fasting schedule, incorporating more physical activity, or reassessing your dietary choices to kickstart your progress and break through the plateau.

Cravings: Cravings are a normal part of the fasting process, but they can be challenging to manage. Experiment with distraction techniques, such as engaging in a hobby or activity, drinking water, or practicing mindfulness exercises, to redirect your focus and overcome cravings without giving in to temptation.

Fatigue: Feeling tired or fatigued during fasting can be a sign that your body needs additional rest or nourishment. Prioritize adequate sleep, hydration, and nutrient-rich foods during your eating windows to support your energy levels and overall well-being.

Hunger: It's natural to experience hunger pangs during fasting, especially when you're first starting out. Remind yourself that hunger is temporary and often subsides after a few minutes. Experiment with hunger management strategies, such as drinking herbal tea, practicing deep breathing exercises, or consuming low-calorie, nutrient-dense snacks, to help curb hunger and stay on track with your fasting goals.

Mindset: Your mindset plays a crucial role in your fasting journey's success. Cultivate a positive and resilient mindset by focusing on progress rather than perfection, practicing self-compassion and patience, and reframing setbacks as opportunities for growth and learning. Trust in your ability to adapt and adjust your approach as needed, and remember that consistency and perseverance are key to achieving long-term success.

By troubleshooting challenges and adjusting your approach with a flexible and proactive mindset, you'll navigate obstacles more effectively and maintain momentum on your fasting journey.

PART SIX

You Are What You Eat

Breakfast, Lunch, Dinner, and Snacks Ideas

In life, we often hear the saying, "You are what you eat." But what does it really mean? Is it just a saying or is there some truth behind it? Let's take a closer look at how the food we eat affects our bodies and why it's important to make healthy choices.

Firstly, let's talk about what it means to be "what you eat." Essentially, this phrase suggests that the food we consume plays a significant role in shaping who we are physically, mentally, and emotionally. Imagine your body as a machine, and the food you eat as the fuel that powers it. Just like a car needs the right type of fuel to run smoothly, our bodies need the right nutrients to function properly.

When we eat nutritious foods like fruits, vegetables, whole grains, and lean proteins, our bodies receive the vitamins, minerals, and other essential nutrients they need to perform various functions. These nutrients help support our immune system, promote healthy growth and development, and even regulate our mood and emotions.

On the other hand, if we consistently consume unhealthy foods like processed snacks, sugary drinks, and fast food, our bodies may not get the nutrients they need to thrive. Instead, we may experience negative effects such as weight gain, fatigue, and an increased risk of developing chronic diseases like diabetes and heart disease.

Now, let's delve into some specific ways that the food we eat can impact our health:

Physical Health: The foods we eat can have a direct impact on our physical health. For example, a diet high in fruits and vegetables can help lower the risk of obesity, high blood pressure, and certain types of cancer. On the other hand, a diet high in processed foods and sugary drinks can contribute to weight gain and increase the risk of developing conditions like diabetes and heart disease.

Mental Health: Believe it or not, what we eat can also affect our mental health. Research has shown that a balanced diet rich in fruits, vegetables, whole grains, and healthy fats can help improve mood and reduce the risk of depression and anxiety. On the flip side, diets high in processed foods and refined sugars have been linked to increased rates of depression and other mental health disorders.

Energy Levels: Have you ever noticed how you feel sluggish and tired after eating a heavy, greasy meal? That's because certain foods can affect our energy levels. Foods high in sugar and refined carbohydrates can cause blood sugar spikes and crashes, leading to feelings of fatigue and lethargy. On the other hand, foods rich in protein, fiber, and healthy fats can provide sustained energy and keep us feeling full and satisfied for longer periods.

Digestive Health: Our digestive system plays a crucial role in breaking down the foods we eat and absorbing nutrients from them. A diet high in fiber from fruits, vegetables, and whole grains can help promote healthy digestion and prevent issues like constipation and bloating. On the other hand, a diet low in fiber and high in processed foods can lead to digestive problems and discomfort.

Long-Term Health: Making healthy food choices isn't just important for our immediate well-being; it also has long-term implications for our overall health and longevity. Research has shown that a nutritious diet can help reduce the risk of chronic diseases like heart disease, stroke, and certain types of cancer. By eating a balanced diet and maintaining a healthy weight, we can increase our chances of living a longer, healthier life.

Now that we understand the importance of making healthy food choices, let's talk about some practical tips for incorporating nutritious foods into our diets:

Consume a Lot of Fruits and veggies: At each meal, try to have half of your plate full of fruits and veggies. These foods are high in antioxidants, vitamins, and minerals—all of which are necessary for optimal health.

Choose Whole Grains: opt for whole grains like brown rice, quinoa, and whole wheat bread instead of refined grains like white rice and white bread. Whole grains are a better option since they contain more fiber and minerals.

Include Lean Proteins: Incorporate lean proteins like chicken, fish, tofu, and beans into your meals. Protein is important for building and repairing tissues and can help keep you feeling full and satisfied.

Limit Processed Foods: Try to limit your intake of processed foods like chips, cookies, and sugary cereals. These foods are often high in unhealthy fats, sugars, and additives that can negatively impact your health.

Drink Plenty of Water: Stay hydrated by drinking plenty of water throughout the day Digestion, vitamin absorption, and general health all depend on water.

Exercise Portion Control: Pay attention to serving sizes and refrain from overindulging. Eating smaller, more frequent meals can help prevent overeating and promote better digestion.

Plan: Give your meals and snacks some thought beforehand. This can help you make healthier choices and avoid impulse eating unhealthy foods.

Listen to Your Body: Observe your feelings in relation to various foods. If certain foods make you feel tired, bloated, or uncomfortable, consider reducing or eliminating them from your diet.

Portion Control and How to Achieve It

The saying "You are what you eat" holds true in many ways. The food we consume has a direct impact on our physical, mental, and emotional well-being. By making healthy food choices and nourishing our bodies with nutritious foods, we can improve our health, increase our energy levels, and live longer, happier lives. So, remember to choose your foods wisely and fuel your body with the nutrients it needs to thrive.

In the world of eating, portion control is a big deal. It's all about how much food you put on your plate and how much you eat. But why is it so important? Well, let's talk about it.

What is Portion Control?

Portion control is all about eating the right amount of food for your body. It means not eating too much or too little. Just the right amount. When you have good portion control, you're giving your body the fuel it needs without overloading it with extra calories.

Why Portion Control is Important

Portion control is important for a few reasons. It first aids in keeping you at a healthy weight. When you eat too much, you're taking in more calories than your body needs. Over time, this may result in weight increase. On the other hand, when you eat too little, you might not be getting enough nutrients to keep your body healthy.

Second, portion control can help prevent overeating. When you eat large portions, it's easy to lose track of how much you're eating. This can lead to mindless eating and consuming more calories than you realize. By controlling your portions, you can avoid this trap and stay on track with your health goals.

Third, portion control can help you manage your blood sugar levels. When you eat large portions of high-carb foods, like pasta or bread, it can cause your blood sugar to spike. This can be especially problematic for people with diabetes or insulin resistance. By keeping your portions in check, you can better regulate your blood sugar and prevent spikes and crashes throughout the day.

How to Achieve Portion Control

Now that we know why portion control is important, let's talk about how to achieve it. Here are a few easy pointers to get you going:

Use Smaller Plates and Bowls: When you use smaller plates and bowls, it can trick your brain into thinking you're eating more than you are. This can assist you in feeling full on lesser servings.

Measure Your Food: Sometimes it's hard to know how much food you're eating. By measuring your portions with cups, spoons, or a food scale, you can get a better idea of how much you should be eating.

Fill Half Your Plate with Veggies: Vegetables are low in calories and high in nutrients, making them the perfect addition to any meal. By filling half your plate with veggies, you can naturally reduce the portion sizes of higher-calorie foods like meats and grains.

Engage in Mindful Eating: by being aware of your body's signals of hunger and fullness. Chew slowly, enjoying every taste. Eat until you're full, not until you're overstuffed.

Plan Your Meals and Snacks: Plan out your meals and snacks ahead of time so you're less likely to overeat. Pack healthy snacks like fruits, nuts, or yogurt to have on hand when hunger strikes.

Avoid Eating Straight from the Package: When you eat straight from the package, it's easy to lose track of how much you're eating. Instead, portion out your food onto a plate or into a bowl so you can see exactly how much you're having.

Drink Water Before Meals: Sometimes thirst can masquerade as hunger. A glass of water before meals can help you feel fuller and avoid overindulging.

Be Mindful of Restaurant Portions: Restaurant portions tend to be larger than what you would serve yourself at home. Consider splitting a meal with a friend or saving half for later to avoid overeating.

Practice Moderation, Not Deprivation: Portion control is all about balance. You don't have to deprive yourself of your favorite foods, but you should enjoy them in moderation.

One of the key components of a healthy diet is portion control. By controlling your portions, you can maintain a healthy weight, prevent overeating, and manage your blood sugar levels. With simple strategies like using smaller plates, measuring your food, and practicing mindful eating, you can achieve portion control and improve your overall health. So next time you sit down to eat, remember to keep your portions in check and listen to your body's cues. Your health will thank you for it.

4 Weeks Breakfast Ideas for Intermittent Fasting

Greek Yogurt Parfait:

Ingredients:
1 cup Greek yogurt,
1/2 cup mixed berries,
1 tablespoon honey,
2 tablespoons granola

Preparation:
In a glass, arrange Greek yogurt, granola, honey, and mixed berries.

Avocado Toast:

Ingredients:
1 slice whole grain bread,
 1/2 avocado,
1 poached egg, salt, pepper, red pepper flakes (optional)

Preparation:
Toast bread, mash avocado on top, add poached egg, season with salt, pepper, and red pepper flakes if desired.

Omelet with Spinach and Feta:

Ingredients:
2 eggs,

1 cup fresh spinach,
1/4 cup crumbled feta cheese, salt, pepper.

Preparation:
Whisk eggs, pour into a heated skillet, add spinach and feta, cook until set.

Chia Seed Pudding:

Ingredients:
2 tablespoons chia seeds,
1 cup unsweetened almond milk,
1/2 teaspoon vanilla extract,
1 tablespoon maple syrup,
1/4 cup sliced strawberries.

Preparation:
Combine almond milk, maple syrup, vanilla essence, and chia seeds. Let sit in the fridge overnight. Serve topped with sliced strawberries.

Whole Grain Pancakes:

Ingredients:
1/2 cup whole wheat flour,
1/2 teaspoon baking powder,
1/2 cup almond milk,
1 egg,
1/2 teaspoon vanilla extract,
1 tablespoon maple syrup

Preparation:

Mix all ingredients, cook pancakes on a heated skillet until golden brown.

Smoothie Bowl:

Ingredients:
 1 frozen banana,
 1/2 cup frozen mixed berries,
 1/2 cup spinach,
 1/2 cup almond milk,
 2 tablespoons granola,
 1 tablespoon almond butter

Preparation:
Blend banana, berries, spinach, and almond milk until smooth. Pour into a bowl, top with granola and almond butter.

Egg Muffins:

Ingredients:
 6 eggs,
 1/2 cup diced bell peppers,
 1/4 cup diced onions,
 1/4 cup chopped spinach,
 1/4 cup shredded cheese,
 salt,
 pepper

Preparation:
Whisk eggs, mix in vegetables and cheese, pour into muffin tin, bake at 350°F (175°C) for 20 minutes.

Quinoa Breakfast Bowl:

Ingredients:
1/2 cup cooked quinoa,
 1/4 cup almond milk,
1 tablespoon honey,
1/4 cup sliced almonds,
1/2 cup mixed berries
Preparation:
 Mix quinoa with almond milk and honey, top with sliced almonds and mixed berries.

Overnight Oats:

Ingredients:
1/2 cup rolled oats,
1/2 cup almond milk,
 1 tablespoon chia seeds,
1 tablespoon maple syrup,
1/4 cup sliced bananas

Preparation:
Mix oats, almond milk, chia seeds, and maple syrup. Let sit in the fridge overnight. Serve topped with sliced bananas.

Egg and Avocado Breakfast Burrito:

Ingredients:
1 whole wheat tortilla,
1 scrambled egg,
1/4 avocado,
salsa,

salt,
pepper

Preparation:
Fill tortilla with scrambled egg, avocado slices, salsa, salt, and pepper. Roll up and serve.

Yogurt and Fruit Bowl:

Ingredients:
1 cup plain yogurt,
1/2 cup sliced strawberries,
1/4 cup blueberries,
1 tablespoon honey,
2 tablespoons chopped nuts (e.g., almonds, walnuts)

Preparation:
Place yogurt in a bowl, top with sliced strawberries, blueberries, honey, and chopped nuts.

Smoked Salmon Bagel:

Ingredients:
1 whole grain bagel,
2 oz smoked salmon,
 2 tablespoons cream cheese,
sliced cucumber,
sliced tomato,
red onion

Preparation:
Toast bagel, spread cream cheese on each half, layer with smoked salmon, cucumber, tomato, and red onion slices.

Green Smoothie:

Ingredients:
1 cup spinach,
1/2 cup frozen pineapple chunks,
1/2 cup frozen mango chunks,
1/2 banana,
1 cup coconut water

Preparation:
Blend spinach, pineapple, mango, banana, and coconut water until smooth.

Egg and Veggie Breakfast Wrap:

Ingredients:
1 whole wheat wrap,
2 eggs,
1/4 cup diced bell peppers,
 1/4 cup diced onions,
1/4 cup chopped spinach,
2 tablespoons shredded cheese,
salt,
pepper

Preparation:
Scramble eggs with bell peppers, onions, and spinach. Fill wrap with scrambled eggs and cheese, season with salt and pepper, and roll up.

Cottage Cheese Bowl:

Ingredients:
1/2 cup cottage cheese,
1/2 cup sliced peaches (fresh or canned in juice),
1 tablespoon honey,
1 tablespoon slivered almonds

Preparation:
Place cottage cheese in a bowl, top with sliced peaches, drizzle with honey, and sprinkle with slivered almonds.

Banana Nut Overnight Oats:

Ingredients:
1/2 cup rolled oats,
1/2 cup almond milk,
1/2 banana (mashed),
1 tablespoon maple syrup,
1 tablespoon chopped walnuts

Preparation:
Mix oats, almond milk, mashed banana, maple syrup, and chopped walnuts. Let sit in the fridge overnight.

Mediterranean Breakfast Plate:

Ingredients:
1 whole wheat pita bread,
 2 tablespoons hummus,
1 hard-boiled egg,
cherry tomatoes,
 cucumber slices,
 olives

Preparation:
Serve pita bread with hummus, sliced hard-boiled egg, cherry tomatoes, cucumber slices, and olives.

Fruit and Nut Toast:

Ingredients:
1 slice whole grain bread,
 2 tablespoons almond butter,
1/2 apple (sliced), 1 tablespoon raisins,
 1 tablespoon chopped almonds

Preparation:
Toast bread, spread almond butter on top, layer with apple slices, raisins, and chopped almonds.

Spinach and Mushroom Frittata:

Ingredients:
4 eggs,
1 cup fresh spinach,
1/2 cup sliced mushrooms,

1/4 cup shredded cheese,
salt,
pepper

Preparation:
Whisk eggs, mix in spinach, mushrooms, and cheese. Pour into a heated skillet and cook until set.

Peanut Butter Banana Smoothie:

Ingredients:
1 banana,
2 tablespoons peanut butter,
1 cup almond milk,
1 tablespoon honey,
1/2 cup ice cubes

Preparation:
Blend banana, peanut butter, almond milk, honey, and ice cubes until smooth.

Tofu Scramble:

Ingredients:
150g firm tofu,
1/4 cup diced bell peppers,
1/4 cup diced onions,
1/4 cup chopped spinach,
1/2 teaspoon turmeric,
salt,
pepper

Preparation:
Crumble tofu into a skillet, add bell peppers, onions, spinach, turmeric, salt, and pepper. Cook until vegetables are tender.

Coconut Chia Pudding:

Ingredients:
1/4 cup chia seeds,
1 cup coconut milk,
1 tablespoon maple syrup,
1/4 teaspoon vanilla extract,
 shredded coconut (for topping)

Preparation:
 Mix chia seeds, coconut milk, maple syrup, and vanilla extract. Refrigerate for a minimum of thirty minutes or for the entire night. Top with shredded coconut before serving.

Breakfast Burrito Bowl:

Ingredients:
1/2 cup cooked quinoa,
1/4 cup black beans,
1 scrambled egg,
1/4 avocado (sliced),
salsa,
cilantro

Preparation:
Layer cooked quinoa, black beans, scrambled egg, sliced avocado, salsa, and cilantro in a bowl.

Blueberry Almond Butter Smoothie:

Ingredients:
1/2 cup frozen blueberries,
1 tablespoon almond butter,
 1/2 cup Greek yogurt,
1/2 cup almond milk,
1 tablespoon honey

Preparation:
Blend blueberries, almond butter, Greek yogurt, almond milk, and honey until smooth.

Vegetable Breakfast Casserole:

Ingredients:
4 eggs,
1 cup diced bell peppers,
1 cup diced onions,
1 cup diced tomatoes,
1 cup chopped spinach,
 1/2 cup shredded cheese,
salt,
pepper

Preparation:
 Whisk eggs, mix in bell peppers, onions, tomatoes, spinach, cheese, salt, and pepper. Pour into a greased baking dish and bake at 375°F (190°C) for 25-30 minutes.

Peanut Butter Banana Overnight Oats:

Ingredients:
1/2 cup rolled oats,
1/2 cup almond milk,
1 tablespoon peanut butter,
1/2 banana (sliced),
1 tablespoon honey

Preparation:
Mix oats, almond milk, peanut butter, banana slices, and honey. Let sit in the fridge overnight.

Breakfast Quinoa Bowl:

Ingredients:
1/2 cup cooked quinoa,
1/4 cup sliced almonds,
1/4 cup dried cranberries,
1/2 teaspoon cinnamon,
1/2 cup almond milk
Preparation:
Mix cooked quinoa, sliced almonds, dried cranberries, cinnamon, and almond milk. Heat until warm.

Egg and Cheese Breakfast Sandwich:

Ingredients:
1 whole grain English muffin,
1 scrambled egg,
1 slice cheese, spinach leaves,

sliced tomato

Preparation:
Toast English muffin, fill with scrambled egg, cheese slice, spinach leaves, and tomato slices.

Chia Seed Breakfast Bowl:

Ingredients:
1/4 cup chia seeds,
1 cup almond milk,
1/2 teaspoon vanilla extract,
1 tablespoon honey,
 sliced strawberries,
sliced banana.

Preparation:
Mix chia seeds, almond milk, vanilla extract, and honey. Let sit in the fridge for at least 30 minutes or until thickened. Top with sliced strawberries and banana.

Mushroom and Spinach Breakfast Quesadilla:

Ingredients:
2 whole wheat tortillas,
1/2 cup sliced mushrooms,
1 cup chopped spinach,
1/4 cup shredded cheese

Preparation:
Heat tortillas in a skillet, top one tortilla with mushrooms, spinach, and cheese. Place the other tortilla on top. Cook until cheese is melted, and tortillas are golden brown.

Protein Pancakes:

Ingredients:
1/2 cup oats,
1/2 cup cottage cheese,
2 eggs,
1/2 teaspoon vanilla extract,
1/2 teaspoon cinnamon

Preparation:
Blend oats, cottage cheese, eggs, vanilla extract, and cinnamon until smooth. Cook on a heated skillet until golden brown on both sides.

Breakfast Stuffed Sweet Potato:

Ingredients:
1 medium sweet potato,
2 tablespoons almond butter,
1 tablespoon honey, 1/4 cup granola,
sliced bananas.

Preparation:
Bake sweet potato until tender. Slice it open and stuff with almond butter, honey, granola, and sliced bananas

4 Weeks Lunch Ideas for Intermittent Fasting

Grilled Chicken Salad:

Ingredients:
4 oz grilled chicken breast,
mixed salad greens,
cherry tomatoes,
cucumber slices,
balsamic vinaigrette

Preparation:
Grill chicken breast, chop vegetables, toss together with vinaigrette.

Quinoa Veggie Bowl:

Ingredients:
1/2 cup cooked quinoa,
roasted vegetables (e.g., bell peppers, zucchini, carrots),
 chickpeas,
feta cheese,
lemon tahini dressing

Preparation:
Cook quinoa, roast vegetables, mix with chickpeas, feta cheese, and drizzle with lemon tahini dressing.

Turkey and Avocado Wrap:

Ingredients:
Whole wheat wrap,
 3 oz sliced turkey breast,
 1/4 avocado,
lettuce,
tomato,
mustard

Preparation:
Fill wrap with turkey, avocado, lettuce, tomato, and mustard. Roll up and serve.

Caprese Salad:

Ingredients:
Fresh mozzarella cheese,
 sliced tomatoes,
fresh basil leaves,
 balsamic glaze,
olive oil,
 salt, pepper

Preparation:
Arrange mozzarella, tomatoes, and basil on a plate. Drizzle with balsamic glaze, olive oil, and season with salt and pepper.

Vegetable Stir-Fry:

Ingredients:
Mixed stir-fry vegetables (e.g., broccoli, bell peppers, snap peas, carrots),
 tofu or chicken,
soy sauce,
garlic,
ginger
Preparation:
Stir-fry vegetables and protein with soy sauce, garlic, and ginger until tender.

Mediterranean Chickpea Salad:

Ingredients:
 Canned chickpeas,
 diced cucumbers,
cherry tomatoes,
Kalamata olives,
feta cheese,
lemon juice,
olive oil,
 oregano

Preparation:
 Rinse chickpeas, mix with vegetables, olives, and feta cheese. Dress with lemon juice, olive oil, and oregano.

Salmon and Asparagus Foil Packets:

Ingredients:
4 oz salmon fillet,
asparagus spears,
lemon slices,
garlic,
olive oil,
salt, pepper

Preparation:
Place salmon and asparagus on foil, season with garlic, olive oil, lemon slices, salt, and pepper. Seal and bake in the oven.

Black Bean Quesadilla:

Ingredients:
Whole wheat tortilla,
black beans,
shredded cheese,
diced bell peppers,
salsa

Preparation:
Fill tortilla with black beans, cheese, and bell peppers. Fold in half and cook until cheese melts. Serve with salsa.

Greek Chicken Pita:

Ingredients:
Whole wheat pita bread,
grilled chicken strips,
 diced tomatoes,
cucumbers,
 red onions,
tzatziki sauce

Preparation:
Fill pita bread with grilled chicken, tomatoes, cucumbers, onions, and tzatziki sauce.

Veggie and Hummus Wrap:

Ingredients:
Whole wheat wrap,
hummus,
sliced bell peppers,
cucumber strips,
shredded carrots,
lettuce

Preparation:
Spread hummus on wrap, layer with vegetables and lettuce. Roll up and enjoy.

Tuna Salad Lettuce Wraps:

Ingredients:
Canned tuna,
Greek yogurt,
diced celery,
diced red onion,
lemon juice,
salt,
 pepper,
lettuce leaves

Preparation:
Mix tuna with Greek yogurt, celery, red onion, lemon juice, salt, and pepper. Serve scoops of tuna salad in lettuce leaves.

Vegetable and Lentil Soup:

Ingredients:
Lentils,
diced tomatoes,
chopped carrots,
chopped celery,
vegetable broth,
garlic,
onion,
spinach,
cumin,
salt,
 pepper

Preparation:
Cook lentils in vegetable broth with tomatoes, carrots, celery, garlic, onion, and spices until tender. Add spinach before serving.

Turkey and Hummus Wrap:

Ingredients:
Whole wheat wrap,
sliced turkey breast,
hummus,
 sliced cucumber,
shredded lettuce,
grated carrots.

Preparation:

Spread hummus on wrap, layer with turkey, cucumber, lettuce, and carrots. Roll up and enjoy.

Quinoa Salad with Chickpeas and Feta:

Ingredients:
 Cooked quinoa,
canned chickpeas,
 diced cucumber,
 cherry tomatoes,

crumbled feta cheese,
lemon juice,
olive oil,
salt,
pepper

Preparation:
Mix quinoa with chickpeas, cucumber, tomatoes, and feta cheese. Add salt, pepper, olive oil, and lemon juice to the dressing.

Egg Salad Sandwich:

Ingredients:
Hard-boiled eggs,
 Greek yogurt,
 diced celery,
 diced red onion,
mustard,
salt,
 pepper,
whole grain bread
Preparation:
Chop hard-boiled eggs and mix with Greek yogurt, celery, red onion, mustard, salt, and pepper. Serve on whole grain bread.

Asian Noodle Salad:

Ingredients:
cooked noodles, like rice or soba noodles,
shredded cabbage,
shredded carrots,
 edamame,
 sliced bell peppers,
 sesame ginger dressing
Preparation:
Toss cooked noodles with vegetables and edamame. Dress with sesame ginger dressing.

Mediterranean Wrap:

Ingredients:
Whole wheat wrap,
hummus,
sliced roasted red peppers,
sliced cucumbers,
crumbled feta cheese,
spinach leaves

Preparation:
Spread hummus on wrap, layer with roasted red peppers, cucumbers, feta cheese, and spinach leaves. Roll up and enjoy.

Chicken Caesar Salad:

Ingredients:

Grilled chicken breast, romaine lettuce,
cherry tomatoes,
grated Parmesan cheese,
Caesar dressing,
croutons

Preparation:
Toss romaine lettuce with sliced grilled chicken, cherry tomatoes, Parmesan cheese, Caesar dressing, and croutons.

Vegetarian Rice Paper Rolls:

Ingredients:
Rice paper wrappers,
shredded lettuce,
sliced cucumber,
shredded carrots,
 sliced avocado,
tofu strips,
hoisin sauce

Preparation:
Dip rice paper wrappers in warm water to soften. Fill with lettuce, cucumber, carrots, avocado, and tofu strips. Roll up and serve with hoisin sauce for dipping.

Mango Black Bean Quinoa Salad:

Ingredients:
Cooked quinoa,
canned black beans,
diced mango,
diced red bell pepper,
diced red onion,
cilantro,
lime juice,
olive oil,
salt,
pepper

Preparation:

Mix quinoa with black beans, mango, bell pepper, red onion, and clantro. Dress with lime juice, olive oil, salt, and pepper.

Greek Orzo Salad:

Ingredients:
Cooked orzo pasta,
diced cucumber,
cherry tomatoes,
Kalamata olives,
crumbled feta
cheese,
red onion,
Greek vinaigrette

Preparation:
Toss cooked orzo with cucumber, tomatoes, olives, feta cheese, red onion, and Greek vinaigrette.

Veggie Sushi Rolls:

Ingredients:
Sushi rice,
nori sheets,
sliced cucumber,
sliced avocado,
shredded carrots,
sliced bell pepper,
pickled ginger,
soy sauce,
wasabi

Preparation:
Spread sushi rice on nori sheets, add vegetables, roll tightly, and slice into sushi rolls. Present alongside wasabi, soy sauce, and pickled ginger.

Chicken Caesar Wrap:

Ingredients:
Whole wheat wrap,
grilled chicken strips,
romaine lettuce,
grated Parmesan cheese,
Caesar dressing

Preparation:
Fill wrap with grilled chicken, romaine lettuce, Parmesan cheese, and Caesar dressing. Roll up and enjoy.

Mushroom and Spinach Quesadilla:

Ingredients:
Whole wheat tortilla,
 sautéed mushrooms,
chopped spinach,
 shredded cheese,
 salsa

Preparation:
Fill tortilla with sautéed mushrooms, spinach, and cheese. Fold in half and cook until cheese melts. Serve with salsa.

Thai Peanut Noodle Salad:

Ingredients:
Cooked soba noodles,
shredded cabbage,
 shredded carrots,
sliced bell peppers,
edamame,
chopped peanuts,
Thai peanut dressing

Preparation:
Toss cooked noodles with vegetables, edamame, chopped peanuts, and Thai peanut dressing.

Vegetable Lentil Curry:

Ingredients:
Cooked lentils,
 diced tomatoes,
diced carrots,
diced potatoes,
diced bell peppers,
coconut milk,
curry paste,
 garlic,
ginger,
onion

Preparation:
Sauté garlic, ginger, and onion, add diced vegetables, lentils, coconut milk, and curry paste. Simmer until vegetables are tender.

Tofu and Veggie Stir-Fry:

Ingredients:
Cubed tofu,
mixed stir-fry vegetables,
soy sauce,
garlic,
ginger,
sesame oil

Preparation:
Sauté tofu until golden brown, add vegetables, soy sauce, garlic, ginger, and sesame oil. Cook until vegetables are tender.

Chickpea Salad Sandwich:

Ingredients:
Mashed chickpeas,
 Greek yogurt,
diced celery,
diced red onion,
lemon juice,
Dijon mustard,
salt,
pepper,
 whole grain bread

Preparation:
 Mix mashed chickpeas with Greek yogurt, celery, red onion, lemon juice, mustard, salt, and pepper. Serve on whole grain bread.

Mediterranean Couscous Salad:

Ingredients:
Cooked couscous,
diced cucumbers,
cherry tomatoes,
Kalamata olives,

crumbled feta cheese,
chopped parsley,
lemon vinaigrette

Preparation:
Toss cooked couscous with cucumbers, tomatoes, olives, feta cheese, parsley, and lemon vinaigrette.

Turkey and Veggie Lettuce Wraps:

Ingredients:
Lettuce leaves,
sliced turkey breast,
sliced bell peppers,
sliced cucumber,
shredded carrots,
avocado slices,
hummus

Preparation:
Fill lettuce leaves with turkey, bell peppers, cucumber, carrots, avocado, and hummus. Roll up and enjoy.

Cauliflower Fried Rice:

Ingredients: Riced cauliflower,
mixed vegetables (e.g., peas, carrots, corn),
scrambled egg,
soy sauce,
garlic,

ginger,
sesame oil

Preparation:
Sauté riced cauliflower with mixed vegetables, scrambled egg, soy sauce, garlic, ginger, and sesame oil until heated throug

4 Weeks Dinner Ideas for Intermittent Fasting

Baked Lemon Herb Chicken:

Ingredients:
Chicken breast,
lemon juice,
garlic,
thyme,
rosemary,
olive oil,
salt, pepper

Preparation:
Marinate chicken in lemon juice, garlic, herbs, olive oil, salt, and pepper. Bake until cooked through.

Vegetable Stir-Fry with Tofu:

Ingredients:
Tofu,
mixed stir-fry vegetables,
soy sauce,
garlic,
 ginger,
sesame oil

Preparation:

Sauté tofu and vegetables in soy sauce, garlic, ginger, and sesame oil until vegetables are tender.

Salmon with Roasted Vegetables:

Ingredients:
Salmon fillet,
mixed vegetables (e.g., broccoli, carrots, cauliflower),
olive oil,
garlic powder,
salt,
pepper

Preparation:
Season salmon and vegetables with olive oil, garlic powder, salt, and pepper. Roast until salmon is cooked and vegetables are tender.

Spaghetti Squash with Marinara Sauce:

Ingredients:
Spaghetti squash,
marinara sauce,
Parmesan cheese,
basil

Preparation:
Roast spaghetti squash, scrape out flesh, top with marinara sauce, Parmesan cheese, and basil.

Grilled Steak with Asparagus:

Ingredients:
Steak,
asparagus,
olive oil,
 garlic,
 salt,
pepper

Preparation:
Season steak with olive oil, garlic, salt, and pepper. Add salt, pepper, and olive oil to grilled asparagus.

Chicken and Vegetable Curry:

Ingredients:
Chicken thighs,
mixed vegetables (e.g., bell peppers, peas, carrots),
coconut milk,
curry paste,
 garlic,
 ginger,
onion

Preparation:
Sauté chicken and vegetables with curry paste, garlic, ginger, and onion. Add coconut milk and simmer until chicken is cooked through.

Shrimp and Vegetable Stir-Fry:

Ingredients:
Shrimp,
mixed stir-fry vegetables,
soy sauce,
garlic,
ginger,
sesame oil

Preparation:
Sauté shrimp and vegetables in soy sauce, garlic, ginger, and sesame oil until shrimp are pink and vegetables are tender.

Stuffed Bell Peppers:

Ingredients:
Bell peppers,
quinoa,
black beans,
 corn,
diced tomatoes,
 shredded cheese,
taco seasoning

Preparation:
Cook quinoa and mix with black beans, corn, diced tomatoes, cheese, and taco seasoning. Stuff into bell peppers and bake until peppers are tender.

Vegetable and Bean Chili:

Ingredients:
Mixed beans (e.g., black beans, kidney beans, chickpeas),
diced tomatoes,
mixed vegetables (e.g., bell peppers, onions, carrots),
chili powder,
cumin,
garlic,
onion

Preparation:
Sauté vegetables and garlic, add beans, tomatoes, chili powder, cumin, and simmer until flavors meld.

Baked Cod with Lemon and Herbs:

Ingredients:
Cod fillets,
lemon slices,
garlic,
parsley,
olive oil,
salt,
pepper

Preparation:
Place cod on a baking sheet, top with lemon slices, garlic, parsley, olive oil, salt, and pepper. Bake until fish flakes easily.

Vegetable and Tofu Teriyaki Stir-Fry:

Ingredients:
Tofu,
mixed stir-fry vegetables,
teriyaki sauce,
garlic,
ginger,
sesame oil

Preparation:
Sauté tofu and vegetables in teriyaki sauce, garlic, ginger, and sesame oil until heated through.

Roasted Chicken Thighs with Sweet Potatoes:

Ingredients:
 Chicken thighs,
sweet potatoes,
olive oil,
rosemary,
thyme,
garlic powder,
salt,
pepper

Preparation:

Coat chicken thighs and sweet potatoes with olive oil, herbs, garlic powder, salt, and pepper. Roast until chicken is cooked through and
sweet potatoes are tender.

Eggplant Parmesan:

Ingredients:
Eggplant slices,
marinara sauce,
mozzarella cheese,
Parmesan cheese,
breadcrumbs,
Italian seasoning

Preparation:
Bread eggplant slices with breadcrumbs and Italian seasoning. Bake until crispy. Layer with marinara sauce and cheese. Bake until the cheese is bubbling and melted.

Taco Salad with Ground Turkey:

Ingredients:
Ground turkey,
 lettuce,
diced tomatoes,
black beans,
corn,
avocado slices,
shredded cheese,
salsa,

tortilla chips

Preparation:
Cook ground turkey with taco seasoning. Assemble salad with lettuce, tomatoes, black beans, corn, avocado, cheese, salsa, and crushed tortilla chips.

Stuffed Zucchini Boats:

Ingredients:
Zucchini,
ground beef or turkey,
marinara sauce,
shredded mozzarella cheese,
 Italian seasoning
Preparation:
Scoop out zucchini seeds to form boats. Fill with cooked ground meat, marinara sauce, and cheese. Bake until zucchini is tender and cheese is melted.

Lemon Garlic Shrimp Pasta:

Ingredients:
Shrimp,
whole wheat pasta,
garlic,
lemon juice,
olive oil,
parsley,
 salt,

pepper

Preparation:
Cook pasta according to package instructions. Sauté shrimp with garlic, lemon juice, olive oil, parsley, salt, and pepper. Toss with cooked pasta.

Vegetable and Chickpea Curry:

Ingredients:
Chickpeas,
mixed vegetables (e.g., cauliflower, carrots, peas),
coconut milk,
curry powder,
garlic,
ginger,
onion

Preparation:
Sauté garlic, ginger, and onion. Add mixed vegetables, chickpeas, coconut milk, curry powder, and simmer until vegetables are tender.

Lentil Shepherd's Pie:

Ingredients:
Cooked lentils,
mixed vegetables (e.g., carrots, peas, corn),
mashed potatoes,
onion, garlic,
vegetable broth,

Worcestershire sauce

Preparation:
Sauté onion and garlic. Add cooked lentils, mixed vegetables, vegetable broth, Worcestershire sauce. Add mashed potatoes on top, then bake until golden.

Honey Garlic Glazed Salmon:

Ingredients:
Salmon fillets,
honey,
soy sauce,
garlic,
ginger,
lemon juice,
olive oil

Preparation:
Mix honey, soy sauce, garlic, ginger, lemon juice, and olive oil. Marinate salmon in the mixture. Bake or grill until cooked through.

Vegetable and Tofu Pad Thai:

Ingredients:
Rice noodles,
tofu,
mixed veggies, such as carrots, bell peppers, and bean sprouts,

scrambled egg,
peanuts,
 pad Thai sauce

Preparation:
Cook rice noodles according to package instructions. Sauté
tofu, vegetables, and scrambled egg. Toss with cooked noodles
and pad Thai sauce. Top with peanuts.

Chicken Fajitas:

Ingredients:
Chicken breast,
bell peppers,
onions,
fajita seasoning,
olive oil,
tortillas,
salsa,
guacamole
Preparation:
Sauté sliced chicken, bell peppers, and onions in olive oil
with fajita seasoning. Serve in tortillas with salsa and
guacamole.

Cauliflower Fried Rice with Shrimp:

Ingredients:
Cauliflower rice,
shrimp,
 mixed vegetables (e.g., peas, carrots, corn),

scrambled egg,
soy sauce,
garlic,
ginger,
sesame oil

Preparation:
Sauté shrimp, vegetables, and scrambled egg in garlic, ginger, soy sauce, and sesame oil. Add cauliflower rice and cook until heated through.

Mushroom and Spinach Stuffed Chicken Breast:

Ingredients:
Chicken breast,
mushrooms,
spinach,
garlic,
mozzarella cheese,
olive oil,
salt,
pepper

Preparation:
Sauté mushrooms and spinach with garlic. Cut a slit in chicken breast and stuff with mushroom mixture and mozzarella cheese. Bake until chicken is cooked through.

Vegetarian Chili:

Ingredients:
Mixed beans, such as pinto, black, and kidney beans,

diced tomatoes,
mixed vegetables (e.g., bell peppers, onions, corn),
chili powder,
cumin,
garlic,
onion

Preparation:
Sauté garlic and onion. Add beans, tomatoes, vegetables, chili powder, cumin, and simmer until flavors meld.

Sesame Ginger Tofu Stir-Fry:

Ingredients:
Tofu,
mixed stir-fry vegetables,
soy sauce,
garlic,
ginger,
sesame oil,
sesame seeds

Preparation:
Sauté tofu and vegetables in soy sauce, garlic, ginger, sesame oil, and sesame seeds until heated through.

Pesto Pasta with Cherry Tomatoes and Chicken:

Ingredients:
Whole wheat pasta,

chicken breast,
cherry tomatoes,
pesto sauce,
Parmesan cheese,
basil

Preparation:
Cook pasta according to package instructions. Sauté chicken until cooked through. Toss cooked pasta with pesto, cherry tomatoes, and cooked chicken. Top with Parmesan cheese and basil.

Teriyaki Glazed Salmon with Broccoli:

Ingredients:
Salmon fillets,
broccoli florets,
teriyaki sauce,
garlic,
ginger,
olive oil,
 sesame seeds

Preparation:
Marinate salmon in teriyaki sauce, garlic, ginger, olive oil. Bake until salmon is cooked through. Toss broccoli with salt, pepper, and olive oil. Serve together and sprinkle with sesame seeds.

Black Bean and Corn Quesadillas:

Ingredients:
Whole wheat tortillas,
black beans,
corn,
diced bell peppers,
shredded cheese,
salsa

Preparation:
Fill tortillas with black beans, corn, bell peppers, and cheese. Cook on a skillet until cheese melts. Serve with salsa.

Chicken and Vegetable Teriyaki Stir-Fry:

Ingredients:
Chicken breast,
mixed stir-fry vegetables,
teriyaki sauce,
 garlic,
ginger,
sesame oil

Preparation:
Sauté chicken and vegetables in teriyaki sauce, garlic, ginger, and sesame oil until heated through.

Vegetable and Lentil Stew:

Ingredients:
Lentils,
mixed vegetables (e.g., carrots, celery, potatoes),
diced tomatoes,
vegetable broth,
garlic,
 onion,
thyme,
rosemary

Preparation:
 Sauté garlic and onion. Add lentils, vegetables, diced tomatoes, vegetable broth, thyme, rosemary, and simmer until lentils are tender.

Baked Stuffed Bell Peppers with Quinoa and Black Beans:

Ingredients:
Bell peppers,
cooked quinoa,
black beans,
 diced tomatoes,
corn,
shredded cheese,
taco seasoning

Preparation:

Mix cooked quinoa with black beans, diced tomatoes, corn, cheese, and taco seasoning. Stuff into bell peppers and bake until peppers are tender, and filling is heated through.

4 Weeks Smoothie Ideas for Intermittent Fasting

Banana Berry Blast:
Banana, mixed berries, spinach, almond milk, Greek yogurt, honey.

Tropical Paradise:
Pineapple, mango, banana, coconut milk, spinach, chia seeds.

Green Goddess:
Kale, spinach, cucumbers, green apples, ginger, lemon juice, and coconut water

Chocolate Peanut Butter Power:
Banana, cocoa powder, peanut butter, almond milk, protein powder (optional), ice cubes.

Strawberry Banana Smoothie:
Strawberries, banana, Greek yogurt, almond milk, honey.

Minty Mango Madness:
Mango, spinach, mint leaves, coconut water, lime juice, chia seeds.

Blueberry Bliss:

Blueberries, banana, spinach, almond milk, Greek yogurt, honey.

Peaches and Cream:

Peaches, bananas, Greek yogurt, almond milk, vanilla extract, ice cubes.

Pineapple Coconut Refresher:

Pineapple, coconut milk, spinach, Greek yogurt, honey.

Berry Beet Bonanza:

Mixed berries, beetroot, spinach, almond milk, Greek yogurt, honey.

Orange Creamsicle Delight:

Oranges, bananas, Greek yogurt, almond milk, vanilla extract, ice cubes.

Chocolate Cherry Almond:

Cherries, cocoa powder, almond butter, almond milk, Greek yogurt, honey.

Kiwi Kale Green Smoothie:

Kiwi, kale, cucumber, green apple, lemon juice, coconut water.

Mango Pineapple Paradise:

Mango, pineapple, spinach, coconut water, Greek yogurt, chia seeds.

Raspberry Coconut Cooler:

Raspberries, coconut milk, spinach, Greek yogurt, honey.

Banana Almond Butter Blast:

Banana, almond butter, almond milk, spinach, Greek yogurt, honey.

Watermelon Mint Refresher:

Watermelon, mint leaves, cucumber, lime juice, coconut water.

Peanut Butter Banana Protein Shake:

Banana, peanut butter, protein powder, almond milk, spinach, honey.

Green Apple Pie Smoothie:

Green apple, oats, cinnamon, almond milk, Greek yogurt, honey.

Berry Avocado Dream:

Mixed berries, avocado, spinach, almond milk, Greek yogurt, honey.

Chocolate Avocado Smoothie:

Avocado, cocoa powder, banana, almond milk, spinach, honey.

Pina Colada Smoothie:

Pineapple, coconut milk, banana, spinach, Greek yogurt, honey.

Mango Matcha Madness:

Mango, matcha powder, spinach, almond milk, Greek yogurt, honey.

Cherry Vanilla Delight:

Cherries, vanilla extract, almond milk, spinach, Greek yogurt, honey.

Orange Carrot Zinger:

Oranges, carrots, ginger, coconut water, Greek yogurt, honey.

Berry Banana Blast:

Mixed berries, banana, spinach, almond milk, Greek yogurt, honey.

Chocolate Cherry Protein Shake:

Cherries, cocoa powder, protein powder, almond milk, spinach, honey.

Peach Raspberry Smoothie:

Peaches, raspberries, spinach, almond milk, Greek yogurt, honey.

Mint Chocolate Chip Shake:

Spinach, mint leaves, cocoa powder, banana, almond milk, Greek yogurt, honey.

Tropical Green Smoothie:

Pineapple, mango, spinach, coconut water, Greek yogurt, honey.

Blueberry Kale Powerhouse:

Blueberries, kale, banana, almond milk, Greek yogurt, honey.

4 weeks Snack Ideas for Intermittent Fasting

Apple Slices with Peanut Butter

Greek Yogurt with Berries

Carrot Sticks with Hummus

Trail Mix (nuts, seeds, dried fruit)

Hard-Boiled Eggs

Cottage Cheese with Pineapple

Whole Grain Crackers with Cheese

Edamame

Rice Cakes with Avocado

Celery Sticks with Almond Butter

Cherry Tomatoes with Mozzarella

Almonds

Popcorn (air-popped)

Banana with Almond Butter

Rice Cake with Cottage Cheese and Sliced Strawberries

Dark Chocolate

Greek Yogurt Parfait with Granola

Bell Pepper Slices with Guacamole

Whole Grain Toast with Smashed Avocado

Homemade Energy Balls (dates, nuts, oats)

Frozen Grapes

Seaweed Snacks

Homemade Veggie Chips (kale, sweet potato, zucchini)

Rice Cake with Tuna Salad

Chia Pudding

Turkey Roll-Ups (sliced turkey wrapped around cucumber)

Pistachios

Hummus and Whole Grain Pita

Roasted Chickpeas

Cheese and Whole Grain Crackers

Yogurt-Dipped Strawberries

4 Weeks Meal Plan Template

Day	Breakfast Smoothie	Lunch Idea	Dinner Idea	Snack Idea
1	Banana Berry Blast	Grilled Chicken Salad	Baked Lemon Herb Chicken	Apple Slices with Peanut Butter
2	Tropical Paradise	Quinoa Veggie Bowl	Vegetable Stir-Fry with Tofu	Greek Yogurt with Berries
3	Green Goddess	Turkey and Avocado Wrap	Salmon with Roasted Vegetables	Carrot Sticks with Hummus
4	Chocolate Peanut Butter Power	Caprese Salad	Spaghetti Squash with Marinara Sauce	Trail Mix
5	Strawberry Banana Smoothie	Vegetable Stir-Fry	Grilled Steak with Asparagus	Hard-Boiled Eggs
6	Minty Mango Madness	Mediterranean Chickpea Salad	Chicken and Vegetable Curry	Cottage Cheese with Pineapple
7	Blueberry Bliss	Salmon and Asparagus Foil Packets	Shrimp and Vegetable Stir-Fry	Whole Grain Crackers with Cheese
8	Peaches and Cream	Black Bean Quesadilla	Stuffed Bell Peppers	Edamame
9	Pineapple Coconut Refresher	Greek Chicken Pita	Vegetable and Bean Chili	Rice Cakes with Avocado

Day	Breakfast Smoothie	Lunch Idea	Dinner Idea	Snack Idea
10	Berry Beet Bonanza	Veggie and Hummus Wrap	Baked Cod with Lemon and Herbs	Celery Sticks with Almond Butter
11	Orange Creamsicle Delight	Greek Orzo Salad	Eggplant Parmesan	Cherry Tomatoes with Mozzarella
12	Chocolate Cherry Almond	Tuna Salad Lettuce Wraps	Taco Salad with Ground Turkey	Almonds
13	Kiwi Kale Green Smoothie	Vegetable and Lentil Soup	Stuffed Zucchini Boats	Popcorn (air-popped)
14	Mango Pineapple Paradise	Chicken Caesar Salad	Lemon Garlic Shrimp Pasta	Banana with Almond Butter
15	Raspberry Coconut Cooler	Mushroom and Spinach Quesadilla	Vegetable and Tofu Teriyaki Stir-Fry	Rice Cake with Cottage Cheese
16	Banana Almond Butter Blast	Asian Noodle Salad	Lentil Shepherd's Pie	Dark Chocolate
17	Watermelon Mint Refresher	Mediterranean Wrap	Honey Garlic Glazed Salmon	Greek Yogurt Parfait with Granola

Day	Breakfast Smoothie	Lunch Idea	Dinner Idea	Snack Idea
18	Peanut Butter Banana Protein Shake	Mango Matcha Madness	Black Bean and Corn Quesadillas	Bell Pepper Slices with Guacamole
19	Green Apple Pie Smoothie	Mango Black Bean Quinoa Salad	Chicken Fajitas	Whole Grain Toast with Smashed Avocado
20	Berry Banana Blast	Greek Yogurt with Berries	Cauliflower Fried Rice with Shrimp	Homemade Energy Balls (dates, nuts, oats)
21	Chocolate Avocado Smoothie	Orange Carrot Zinger	Mushroom and Spinach Stuffed Chicken Breast	Frozen Grapes
22	Pina Colada Smoothie	Vegetable and Chickpea Curry	Lentil Shepherd's Pie	Seaweed Snacks
23	Blueberry Kale Powerhouse	Lentil Shepherd's Pie	Baked Stuffed Bell Peppers	Homemade Veggie Chips (kale, sweet potato, zucchini)
24	Mango Pineapple Paradise	Honey Garlic Glazed Salmon	Teriyaki Glazed	Rice Cake with Tuna Salad

Day	Breakfast Smoothie	Lunch Idea	Dinner Idea	Snack Idea
			Salmon with Broccoli	
25	Strawberry Banana Smoothie	Pesto Pasta with Cherry Tomatoes	Black Bean and Corn Quesadillas	Chia Pudding
26	Mint Chocolate Chip Shake	Peach Raspberry Smoothie	Chicken and Vegetable Teriyaki Stir-Fry	Turkey Roll-Ups (sliced turkey wrapped around cucumber or avocado)
27	Tropical Green Smoothie	Mint Chocolate Chip Shake	Vegetable and Lentil Stew	Pistachios
28	Chocolate Cherry Protein Shake	Berry Avocado Dream	Sesame Ginger Tofu Stir-Fry	Hummus and Whole Grain Pita
29	Green Goddess	Orange Creamsicle Delight	Pina Colada Smoothie	Roasted Chickpeas
30	Mango Matcha Madness	Chocolate Peanut Butter Power	Blueberry Kale Powerhouse	Cheese and Whole Grain Crackers
31	Banana Berry Blast	Green Apple Pie Smoothie	Chocolate Avocado Smoothie	Yogurt-Dipped Strawberries

CONCLUSION

Your Journey Ahead: A Final Word

Congratulations! You've reached the end of this journey, and what a journey it has been. As you look ahead to the road that lies before you, there are a few things to keep in mind. Let's wrap up this adventure with some simple but powerful words.

1. Reflect on Your Achievements:

Consider for a moment how far you've come. You've learned so much about intermittent fasting and how it can benefit your health. You've made changes to your lifestyle and habits, and you've seen the results. No matter how modest they may appear, acknowledge and celebrate your accomplishments.

2. Stay Committed to Your Goals:

Now is not the time to rest on your laurels. Keep your eyes on the prize and stay committed to your goals. Whether you're looking to lose weight, improve your health, or just feel better overall, remember why you started this journey in the first place. Keep pushing forward, one step at a time.

3. **Embrace Challenges as Opportunities**:

You can run into difficulties and setbacks along the route. However, don't allow them to demoralize you. Rather, consider them as chances for development and education. Every obstacle you conquer increases your strength and adaptability. With wide arms, welcome them and continue on your way.

4. **Remember to Listen to Your Body:**

Your body is incredibly smart, so be sure to listen to what it's telling you. If you're feeling tired, take a rest. If you're hungry, eat something nutritious. Pay attention to how different foods and fasting schedules affect you and adjust accordingly. Your body knows what it needs, so trust it.

5. **Stay Connected and Supported**:

Remember to rely on your support network as necessary. Assemble a support system of friends, family, and online communities to help and inspire you. Tell them about your triumphs and setbacks and allow them to encourage you to keep moving forward on your path.

6. **Keep Learning and Growing**:

This is just the beginning of your health and wellness journey. Keep seeking out new information, trying new things, and pushing yourself outside of your comfort zone. The more you learn and grow, the better equipped you'll be to navigate the road ahead.

7. **Trust in Yourself:**

Above all else, trust in yourself and your ability to succeed. You've already proven that you're capable of making positive changes in your life. Have faith in your resiliency, resolve, and strength. You have everything you need to create the life you desire.

As you embark on the next phase of your journey, remember these words of wisdom. Stay focused, stay determined, and above all else, stay true to yourself. Your future is bright, and the possibilities are endless. Here's to the incredible adventure that lies ahead. Go forth and conquer.